Our Healthier Nation

A Contract for Health

Presented to Parliament by the Secretary of State for Health

by Command of Her Majesty ~ February 1998

Cm 3852   £10.30

Contents

Foreword - Our Healthier Nation   2

Summary   4

Chapter 1   Fit for the 21st Century   7

Chapter 2   The Causes of Ill Health   15

Chapter 3   A Contract for Health   28

Chapter 4   Targets for Health   55

Chapter 5   Your Views on Better Health   84

Glossary and Technical Notes   86

References   88

Questionnaire: Your Views on Better Health   91

Foreword

Good health. It's not just a toast. It's what everybody wants for themselves, their family and friends. If you are a parent, it's the supreme gift you'd like to give your children. For the sake of every individual, for society and for the economy, it should be a top priority for any Government. It is a top priority for this Government.

While health generally has improved, far too many people are still falling ill and dying sooner than they should. The NHS is there to provide treatment and care when people fall ill. Our recent White Paper - *The new NHS* - spells out our proposals for a modern and dependable health service. But it's not enough to treat people when they fall ill. We've got to do more to stop them falling ill in the first place.

That means tackling the root causes of the avoidable illnesses. In recent times the emphasis has been on trying to get people to live healthy lives, where necessary by changing their lifestyle. Now we want to see far more attention and Government action concentrated on the things which damage people's health which are beyond the control of the individual.

Poor people are ill more often and die sooner. To tackle these fundamental inequalities we must concentrate attention and resources on the areas most affected by air pollution, poverty, low wages, unemployment, poor housing, crime and disorder, which can make people ill in both body and mind.

The new Government is already taking action to tackle all these problems. That will improve the health of the worst off and least healthy people and neighbourhoods.

This Green Paper sets out our proposals for concerted action by the Government as a whole in partnership with local organisations, to improve people's living conditions and health. It recognises that there are limits to what Government can do and spells out what the individual can do, if the Government do their bit. That's why we are proposing a 'contract for health'.

We put forward specific targets for tackling some of the major killer diseases and proposals for local action. But the Government doesn't believe we have a monopoly of concern and knowledge. So we are inviting everyone who is interested to let us have their comments on what we are proposing and to put forward suggestions of their own.

Frank Dobson
Secretary of State for Health

Tessa Jowell
Minister of State for Public Health

Summary

Good health is treasured. It is the foundation of a good life. Better health for the nation is central to making a better country.

'major opportunities to improve people's health'

We have major opportunities to improve people's health. Almost 90,000 people die every year before they reach their 65th birthday. Of these, nearly 32,000 die of cancer, and 25,000 die of heart disease, stroke and related illnesses. Many of these deaths could be prevented.

Health inequalities are widening. The poorest in our society are hit harder than the well off by most of the major causes of death. In improving the health of the whole nation, a key priority will be better health for those who are worst off.

There are sound economic reasons for improving our health. 187 million working days are estimated by industry to be lost every year because of sickness - a £12 billion tax on business.

'sound economic reasons'

Treating ill health is expensive. Heart disease, stroke and related illnesses cost the National Health Service an estimated £3.8 billion every year. By preventing avoidable illness we can concentrate resources on treating conditions which cannot yet be prevented.

Poor health has complex causes. Some are fixed - ageing, for instance, or genetic factors. Our priority is to concentrate on the factors which affect people's health, and on which we can all make an impact.

These include a range of factors to do with how we all live our lives - diet, physical activity, sexual behaviour, smoking, alcohol and drugs.

Social and economic issues play a part too - poverty, unemployment and social exclusion. So too does our environment - air and water quality, and housing. And so does access to good services, like education, transport, social services and the NHS itself.

Tackling these health issues involves a range of linked programmes, including measures on welfare to work, crime, housing and education, as well as on health itself.

In the proposals put forward in this consultative Green Paper, *Our Healthier Nation*, the Government has two key aims:

- To improve the health of the population as a whole by increasing the length of people's lives and the number of years people spend free from illness.

- To improve the health of the worst off in society and to narrow the health gap.

'a third way between the old extremes of individual victim blaming on the one hard and nanny state social engineering on the other'

To achieve these aims, the Government is setting out a third way between the old extremes of individual victim blaming on the one hand and nanny state social engineering on the other.

Good health is no longer about blame, but about opportunity and responsibility.

While people on their own can find it hard to make a difference, when individuals, families, local agencies and communities and the Government work together deep-seated problems can be tackled.

Our third way is a national contract for better health. Under this contract, the Government, local communities and individuals will join in partnership to improve all our health.

'Government, local communities and individuals will join in partnership to improve all our health'

For its part, the Government will help assess the risk to health by making sure that people are given information on health which is accurate, understandable and credible. Where there are real threats to health we will not hesitate to take tough action - though regulation and legislation will be the exception, not the rule.

Health Authorities will have a key role in leading local alliances to develop Health Improvement Programmes, which will identify local needs and translate the national contract into local action.

Local Authorities will have a new duty to promote the economic, social and environmental well-being of their areas.

Businesses can bring new skills to bear, including marketing and communications - as well as improving the health and safety of their own employees.

Voluntary bodies can act as advocates to give a powerful voice to local people.

Individuals can take responsibility for their own health.

To help enact the contract, we have identified three settings for action:

- Healthy schools - focusing on children

- Healthy workplaces - focusing on adults

- Healthy neighbourhoods - focusing on older people

'to make real
progress, we will
focus on four
priority areas'

And to make real progress, we will focus on four priority areas, setting clear targets for improvement in each:

By the year 2010:

- **HEART DISEASE AND STROKE.** **target**: to reduce the death rate from heart disease and stroke and related illnesses amongst people aged under 65 years by at least **a further third**

- **ACCIDENTS**[†]. **target**: to reduce accidents by at least **a fifth**

- **CANCER.** **target**: to reduce the death rate from cancer amongst people aged under 65 years by at least **a further fifth**

- **MENTAL HEALTH.** **target**: to reduce the death rate from suicide and undetermined injury by at least **a further sixth**.

'tough targets...
challenging
targets'

These are tough targets. They are challenging targets. With this consultation paper, we want to know what you think of them. There are strong personal, social and economic arguments for making our health better. This Government intends to act on them.

[†]An accident is defined here as one which involves a hospital visit or consultation with a family doctor.

Fit for the 21st Century

The Case for Health

1.1   There are strong personal, social and economic arguments for making our health better. The Government intends to act on them. We know that progress has been made, but more needs doing. There are still major opportunities to improve our health.

'progress has been made, but more needs doing'

The Personal Case

1.2   Good health is the foundation of a good life. Our own health and the health of our families and friends underpin our ability to enjoy life to the full. When we are well we are able to make the most of the opportunities that life has to offer and to play a full part in family, community and working life. No matter what goes wrong in life - money, work or relationship problems - good health helps sustain us.

'good health is the foundation of a good life'.

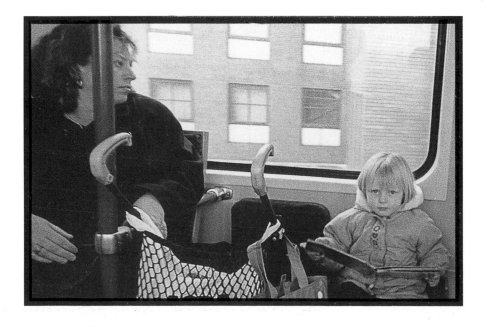

How often have we all heard someone say that although things may not be going well - at least they have their health. Good health is treasured.

1.3   Good health also means not living in fear of illness, constantly worried about our health or the health of those closest to us. It means being confident and positive and able to cope with the ups and downs of life. Better health for the nation is central to making a better country.

1.4   It's good that people are generally living longer and living healthier lives. But the level of illness remains a cause for concern. Estimates based on Government statistics show there are over 250 million visits to GPs and 70 million visits to hospitals every year. Now, in the 1990s, nearly 90,000 people die each year before they reach their 65th birthday. Of these people, more than 25,000 die of heart disease, stroke and related illnesses and 32,000 die of cancer. Many of these deaths could be prevented.

'good health is about quality of life'

1.5   But good health is <u>not</u> just about how long people live. It is also about quality of life and how well people are during those extra years, so that they are not robbed of their dignity and independence in later life. Figure 1 shows that although both men and women are living longer, they spend many of those years in poor health. What we want is a healthier country where people spend as little time as possible burdened by sickness, pain and disability.

**Figure 1.
Life expectancy and healthy life expectancy**

At birth, Great Britain 1994

Source: Bebbington and Darton (1996), from Office for National Statistics (ONS) data.

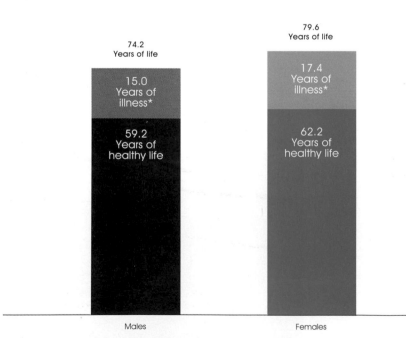

*Limiting long-standing illness - based on a positive response to the following questions in the General Household Survey:
(1) Do you have any long-standing illness, disability or infirmity?
(2) Does the illness or disability limit your activities in any way?

This chart presents Healthy Life Expectancy calculated on the basis of self-reported "limiting long-standing illness". Extra years of life gained over recent years have on the basis of this methodology, been years of mild to moderate disability. Other research however suggests that with respect to measures of more severe disability, healthy life expectancy at age 65 years has shown some improvements alongside total life expectancy. The extra years of life have not therefore been years of severe disability.

The Social Case

1.6   In a modern and strong society, united by core values of fairness and compassion, it is vital that everyone gains from a national drive for better health.

1.7   A healthy country would be one where health was not dictated by accident of birth and childhood experience. Everyone should have a fair chance of a long and healthy life.

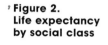

everyone should have a fair chance of a long and healthy life'

1.8   The general improvement in health stems largely from improved living standards. But not all have shared in growing prosperity. Surveys over the last few years have shown a growing gap in wealth between the best and worst off people and the best and worst off neighbourhoods. Predictably the most recent figures[1] from the Office for National Statistics show that the health gap is growing as well.

1.9   The poorest in our society are hit harder than the well off by most of the major causes of death. Poor people are ill more often and die sooner. The life expectancy of those higher up the social scale (in professional and managerial jobs) has improved more than those lower down (in manual and unskilled jobs). This inequality has widened since the early 1980s (see figure 2).

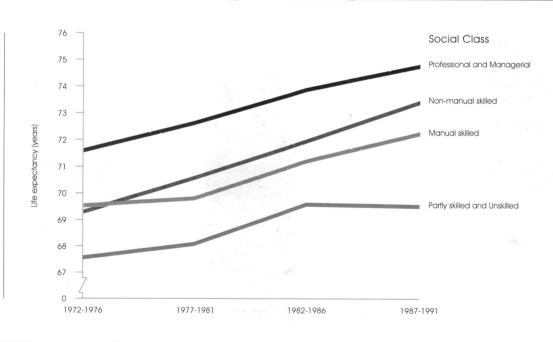

**Figure 2.
Life expectancy
by social class**

Males at birth
England and Wales
1972-1991

Source: adapted from
Drever and Whitehead
(eds), Health Inequalities,
ONS, (1997), using data
from ONS Longitudinal Study

Social Class

Professional and Managerial

Non-manual skilled

Manual skilled

Partly skilled and Unskilled

1.10 In the past this social dimension was frequently neglected. Poor health was put down to bad luck, unhealthy behaviour, or inadequate healthcare.

1.11 Yet it is clear that people's chances of a long and healthy life are basically influenced by how well off they are, where they live and by their ethnic background. A child's chance of surviving to its first birthday relates to the country of birth of its mother, as figure 3 shows. Figure 4 shows how men's social class can influence their chances of dying from lung cancer before the age of retirement. Figure 5 shows how some areas are hit harder by deaths before the age of 65.

Figure 3.
Infant mortality rate*

By mother's country of birth, deaths in England and Wales 1994-1996 combined

*Deaths before age 1 per 1,000 live births.

Source: ONS Monitors DH3 (1995, 1996, 1997).

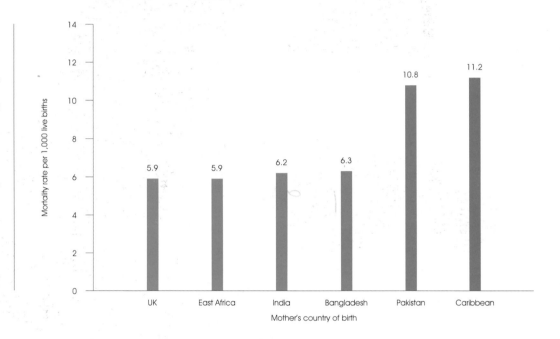

Figure 4.
Mortality from lung cancer by social class

Men, aged 20-64 England and Wales 1991-1993

Source: Drever and Whitehead (eds), Health Inequalities ONS, (1997) using data from death registrations and 1991 Census.

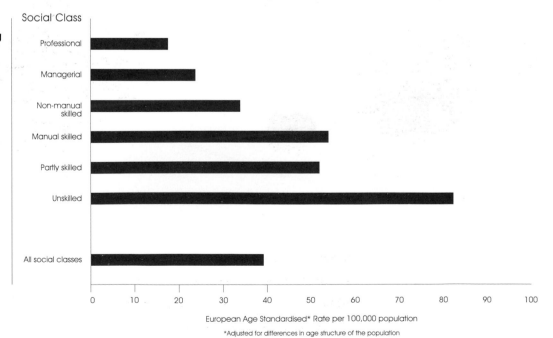

Parts of Tyne Tees, Greater Manchester, the West Midlands and London have some of the highest rates of early death, whilst most of East Anglia and the South West have the lowest.

**Figure 5.
Geographical
inequalities in
mortality**

By Health Authority,
persons aged 15-64
1994-1996

Standardised Mortality
Ratios (SMRs) from all
causes. (see glossary)

Source: Public Health
Common Data Set 1997
(from ONS data),

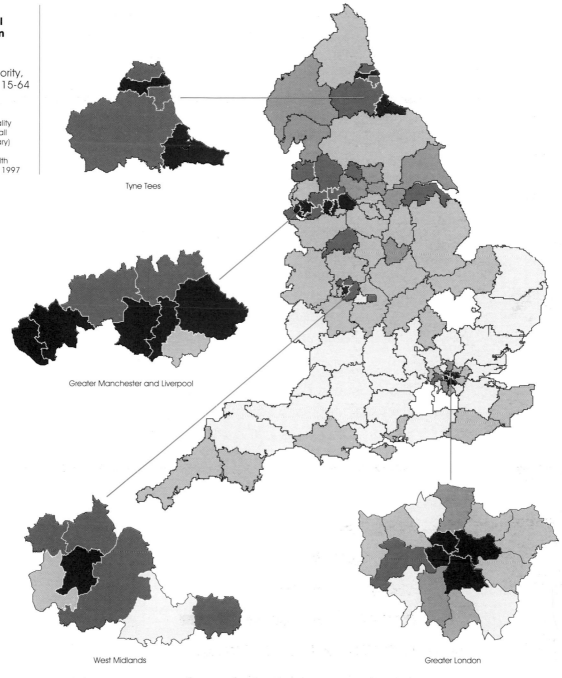

Tyne Tees

Greater Manchester and Liverpool

West Midlands

Greater London

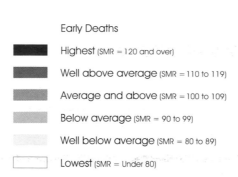

Early Deaths

◼ Highest (SMR = 120 and over)

◼ Well above average (SMR = 110 to 119)

◼ Average and above (SMR = 100 to 109)

◻ Below average (SMR = 90 to 99)

◻ Well below average (SMR = 80 to 89)

◻ Lowest (SMR = Under 80)

1.12 The Government recognises that the social causes of ill health and the inequalities which stem from them must be acknowledged and acted on. **Connected problems require joined-up solutions. This means tackling inequality which stems from poverty, poor housing, pollution, low educational standards, joblessness and low pay. Tackling inequalities generally is the best means of tackling health inequalities in particular**.

'tackling inequalities generally is the best means of tackling health inequalities in particular'

1.13 Within our overall programme to improve the health of the whole population a key priority will be to improve the health of those who are marginalised and worst off. We will seek to improve the absolute and relative positions of those people and areas which are hit hardest by poor health and premature death. That will narrow the gap between them and the better off .

1.14 Moreover, social exclusion can be both a *cause* and an *effect* of ill health. If people are too ill to work or to participate in everyday social life, isolated from the mainstream opportunities by illness or disability, then they can become socially excluded. If they are not in society's mainstream, they are more likely to damage their health by smoking or they may seek comfort in activities like illegal drug-taking and so damage their health.

'to succeed in the modern world economy, the country's workforce must be healthy as well as highly skilled'

The Economic Case

1.15 A healthy population is a key factor in a prosperous and modern economy. There are sound and hard-headed business reasons for making our health better.

1.16 To succeed in the modern world economy, the country's workforce must be healthy as well as highly skilled. The Confederation of British Industry has estimated that 187 million working days are lost each year because of sickness[2]. That's a £12 billion social tax on business every year, damaging to competitiveness and a brake on prosperity.

'by preventing avoidable illnesses we can enable the NHS to concentrate its resources on treating those conditions which cannot yet be prevented'

1.17 Cancer treatments cost the NHS an estimated £1.3 billion each year, whilst heart disease, stroke and related illnesses cost £3.8 billion. Treating accidents and other injuries costs some £1.2 billion and treating poor mental health in excess of £5 billion a year[3]. Illnesses caused by smoking cost the NHS between £1.4 and £1.7 billion each year. By preventing avoidable illnesses we can enable the NHS to concentrate its resources on treating those conditions which cannot yet be prevented.

1.18 Investing in the country's health is partly about working for a fair and decent society. It is partly about using the resources of the health service to best effect. But, equally importantly, it is also part of the

Government's determined drive to improve England's economic efficiency and performance.

Our Health Can Be Better

1.19 Our health today falls short of what we already know is possible. It is better here than in many other European countries. But it is hit harder than some countries by the big killer diseases. And, as figure 6 shows, people in England have less chance of a long life than people living in France, Italy or Sweden.

**Figure 6.
Expectation of life
at birth**

European Union
circa 1995*

*Data for 1995 except for
Austria 1996; Denmark and
France 1994; Ireland, Italy
and Spain 1993; Belgium
1992.

Figures for England
calculated by Government
Actuary's Department, by
slightly different
methodology to WHO
figures, (however this does
not affect the ranking of the
countries).

Source: WHO Health For All
statistical database and
Government Actuary's
Department.

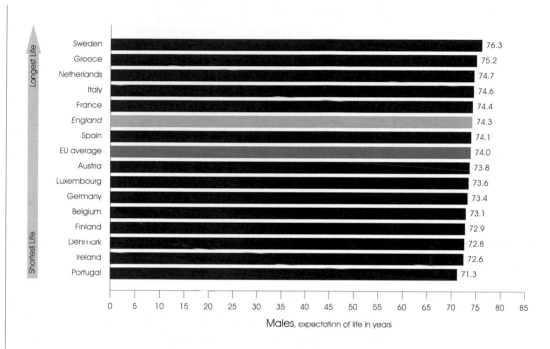

Males, expectation of life in years

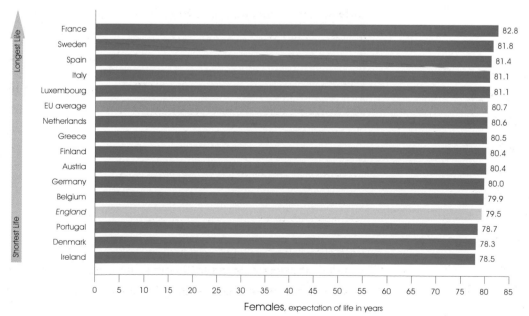

Females, expectation of life in years

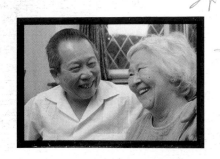

1.20 Compared with other countries, many people - particularly older people - still spend much of their lives in pain or discomfort, dependent on others for support. At a time when they should be free to make the very most of their lives too many spend their retirement unable to enjoy the independence that people who are well take for granted[4]. We want to ensure a more comfortable retirement which gives people the ability to live independently and to do things for themselves for as long as possible.

Our Healthier Nation

1.21 So there is an overwhelming personal, social and economic case, based on common sense, for improving our health. The Government is determined to play its part in a concerted effort to make our health better.

1.22 It is obvious that problems that have persisted for decades will not be solved overnight. The results of our efforts may take years to show through in better health. Improvements in health will not be easy to secure. They will have to happen at a pace which people can accept and which the country can afford. There will be hard choices to be made by us all. But this is no excuse for inactivity and in time our efforts can and will make a real difference.

1.23 The Government has two overriding aims for *Our Healthier Nation*.

> **Our Healthier Nation - Two Key Aims for improving the health of the population**
>
> - *To improve the health of the population as a whole by increasing the length of people's lives and the number of years people spend free from illness.*
>
> - *To improve the health of the worst off in society and to narrow the health gap.*

1.24 The Government has identified four priority areas for action - heart disease and stroke, accidents, cancer and mental health - and proposes to set a national target for each of them. These targets will give purpose and direction to the strategy and help us to assess overall progress.

1.25 This Green Paper sets out the Government's proposals on how, together, we can achieve our two overriding aims, and asks for your views on them. When your views have been taken into account, we will publish later this year a White Paper setting out a strategy for action.

'we want to ensure a more comfortable retirement which gives people the ability to live independently'

'the Government is determined to play its part in a concerted effort to make our health better'

'this Green Paper asks for your views'

The Causes of Ill Health

Understanding the Causes of Ill Health

2.1   Our understanding of how and why people become ill has advanced in leaps and bounds in the past century, with British science and know-how often at the forefront of international efforts. For example, it has played a key role in proving the link between smoking and cancer, in the development of life-saving vaccines and in understanding the factors, such as air pollution, which cause other diseases. British medical science has also played a leading role in developing such treatments as antibiotics, anaesthetics and key-hole surgery. The Government will continue to support this British research. We are determined that this proud history will continue.

2.2   But the causes of ill health are complex. There are still many illnesses which we do not fully understand and which can strike unexpectedly. Some are caused by genetic factors fixed before our birth, some by factors beyond our individual control, and others by the way we live. Whatever the causes of ill health we need a health care system to treat and care for people who fall ill. The Government's renewal of the health service, set out in the White Paper, *The new NHS*[5], will ensure a modern and dependable NHS. This is especially vital for those who are poor or vulnerable, who are likely to have the worst general health and so the greatest need to use the NHS.

2.3   Some of the main factors which influence our health are shown in the table overleaf. This sets out a whole range of factors - those which are beyond the influence of individuals and so require wider national and local efforts to secure progress, alongside those which are determined by individual behaviour.

'the causes of ill health are complex'

'the Government's renewal of the health service, set out in the White Paper, *The new NHS* will ensure a modern and dependable NHS'

Factors affecting health				
Fixed	**Social and Economic**	**Environment**	**Lifestyle**	**Access to Services**
Genes	Poverty	Air quality	Diet	Education
Sex	Employment	Housing	Physical activity	NHS
Ageing	Social exclusion	Water quality	Smoking	Social Services
		Social environment	Alcohol	Transport
			Sexual behaviour	Leisure
			Drugs	

Fixed factors

2.4   Although our age, sex and genetic make-up have a major influence on our health, for most people there is little we can do about them. But we can try to modify some of their predictable consequences. Within a few years we can expect developments in genetic science to make it possible to do much more than we can now.

Social and Economic Factors

Poverty

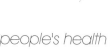

'people's health is affected by their circumstances'

2.5   People's health is affected by their circumstances. Well-being, a sense of control over your life, and optimism about the future is good for health. For example:

- low income can make it hard to afford to keep your house warm or protect yourself and your family from fire and accidents in the home, such as by buying smoke alarms or replacing faulty wiring;

- low income, deprivation and social exclusion all influence smoking levels. It's harder to stop smoking when you're worrying about making ends meet. One study found that while a third of children in the United Kingdom lived with at least one adult smoker, for low income families, the figure rose to 57%[6].

- if the nearest supermarket is miles away or the bus doesn't go there when you can, it can be difficult to buy food which is cheap and healthy;

- if the street outside your home is busy with traffic or there are drug dealers in the park then it's safer to keep the kids in front of the TV than let them out to play.

Employment

2.6   Being in work is good for your health. Joblessness has been clearly linked to poor physical and mental health. Figure 7 shows how those in work tend to live longer lives than those without jobs. Unemployed men and women are more likely than people in work to die from cancer, heart disease, accidents and suicide. Losing his job doubles the chances of a middle-aged man dying within the next five years.

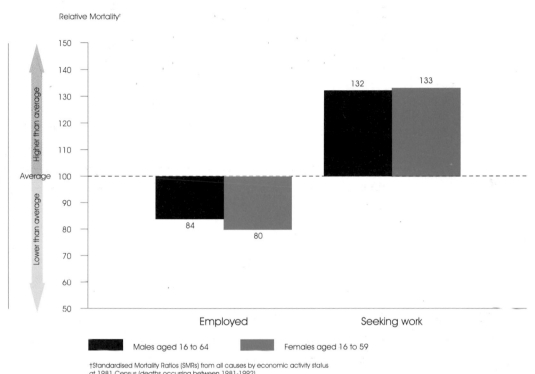

Figure 7. Employment, unemployment* and mortality

By sex, England and Wales 1981-1992

*Unemployment = People currently unemployed but seeking work. The chart does not include those who are permanently sick or disabled, or inactive for other reasons.

Source: Drever and Whitehead (eds), Health Inequalities ONS, (1997) using data from ONS Longitudinal Study.

†Standardised Mortality Ratios (SMRs) from all causes by economic activity status at 1981 Census (deaths occurring between 1981-1992)

Social Exclusion

2.7   When social problems - poor housing, unemployment or low pay, fear of crime and isolation - are combined, as they often are, then people's health can suffer disproportionately. Social exclusion involves not only social but also economic and psychological isolation. Although people may know what affects their health, their hardship and isolation mean that it is often difficult to act on what they know. The best way to make a start on helping them live healthier lives is to provide help and support to enable them to participate in society, and to help them improve their own economic and social circumstances. That will help to improve their health.

'a safe, secure
and sustainable
environment is a
pre-requisite for a
healthy nation'

Environment

2.8   A safe, secure and sustainable environment is a pre-requisite for a healthy nation. The way in which the environment affects our health is sometimes easily explicable but more often involves a complex mix of factors. Such things as clean air and water and good quality housing are important to our health and well-being.

Air Quality

2.9   People need to know that if they don't smoke, or if they are giving up smoking, then the Government, Local Authorities and businesses are also taking action to ensure that general pollution is not harming their health and that the quality of the air they breathe is good. A recent study has suggested that high levels of ozone in the air in the summer months lead to increased hospital admissions for respiratory disorders[7,8].

Housing

2.10 Housing has an important impact on health. Research has shown that the most significant risks from poor housing are associated with damp, which can contribute to diseases of the lungs and other parts of the respiratory system[9,10,11,12]. Cramped living in poor conditions leads to accidents, sleeplessness, stress and the rapid spread of infections.

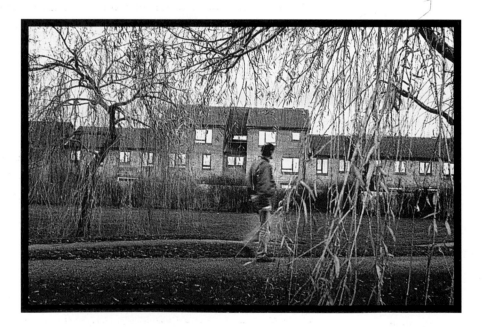

'a million homes
have inadequate
energy efficiency'

2.11 Many deaths each year are due to cold conditions. Older people and the very young are particularly vulnerable to cold weather. About a million homes in the United Kingdom have inadequate standards of energy efficiency, putting the health of those who live in them at risk when it's cold.

2.12 100,000 houses in the United Kingdom have high levels of radon gas. People want to be confident that if they are acting responsibly and protecting themselves from cancer by eating well and not smoking, then the Government and Local Authorities are actively engaged in reducing the health risk in those areas where radon gas in homes can increase the chances of developing lung cancer[13,14].

'families with small children and older people need plentiful supplies of water'

Water Quality

2.13 The quality of the water we drink is an important influence on health. Some of the very earliest public health measures were about tackling water-borne diseases such as cholera. Moreover families with small children and older people need plentiful supplies of water for washing at prices they can afford. The Government will set a stringent standard of 10µg/l to reduce lead in drinking water, as supplied to homes, to be met within 15 years. The Government will also ensure that water suppliers will continue to treat water to reduce its ability to dissolve lead and for most properties this will ensure that levels at the tap - that is after any contamination by the property owner's pipes - do not exceed 25µg/l. The Government will be preparing advice for homeowners to help them take an informed decision on options for action if they have lead pipes within their homes.

2.14 There are many other environmental influences on our health, including noise pollution, global warming, ozone depletion, and carbon monoxide in the home. But there is also the important context of ensuring that particular environments, such as work and the community, are healthy ones.

Social Environment

2.15 The quality of life in the community and the extent to which people respect and support each other can also be important to our health. Social exclusion can have damaging health consequences. One study found that, compared to people with lots of social ties, the socially isolated were over six times more likely to die from a stroke and more than three times more likely to commit suicide[15].

2.16 Neighbourhoods where people know and trust each other and where they have a say in the way the community is run can be a powerful support in coping with the day to day stresses of life which affect health. And having a stake in the local community gives people self-respect and makes them feel better.

'tackling crime and fear of crime in the community can have a direct impact on our health'

2.17 Tackling crime and fear of crime in the community can have a direct impact on our health. Sadly, many people may be afraid to go out for walks alone. They may suffer stress from being victims of crime or from living in an area where crime is commonplace and so they live in fear. Measures to tackle youth crime and develop local crime prevention strategies will help people feel secure in their homes, and reduce some of the stresses in their lives caused by the fear of crime.

Lifestyle

2.18 How people live has an important impact on health. Whether people smoke; whether they are physically active; what and how much they eat and drink; their sexual behaviour and whether they take illicit drugs - all of these factors can have a dramatic and cumulative influence on how healthy people are and how long they will live.

Diet and Physical Activity

'a good diet is an important way of protecting health'

2.19 A good **diet** is an important way of protecting health. The amount of fruit and vegetables people eat is an important influence on health. Unhealthy diets, which tend to include too much sugar, salt and fatty foods, are linked to cancer, heart disease and stroke as well as tooth decay[16,17]. Research suggests that a third of all cancers are the result of a poor diet[18]. The amount of **physical activity** that people take is also an important factor in preventing heart disease, building healthy bones and helping to maintain good mental health.

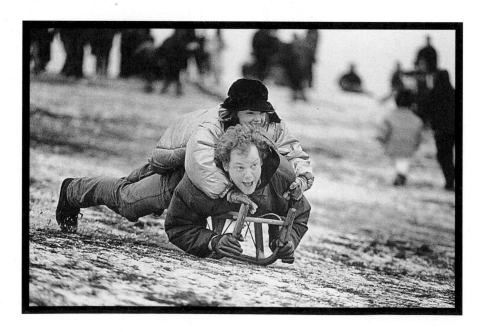

'smoking is estimated to account for nearly a fifth of all deaths each year'

Smoking

2.20 **Smoking** is the biggest cause of diseases which lead to early deaths in England. It is estimated to account for nearly a fifth of all deaths each year - 120,000 lives in the United Kingdom cut short or taken by tobacco[19]. Smoking is the main cause of lung cancer and is linked to heart disease, chronic bronchitis, asthma and cancers of the mouth, bladder, kidney, stomach and pancreas. Mothers who smoke increase the risk of cot deaths to their babies[20]. Figure 8 shows the range of risks that smokers face.

**Figure 8.
The health risks of cigarette smoking**

Source: based on Smoke-free for Health, DOH (1994), from US Office on Smoking and Health, Centers for Disease Control and Prevention Report, (1990).

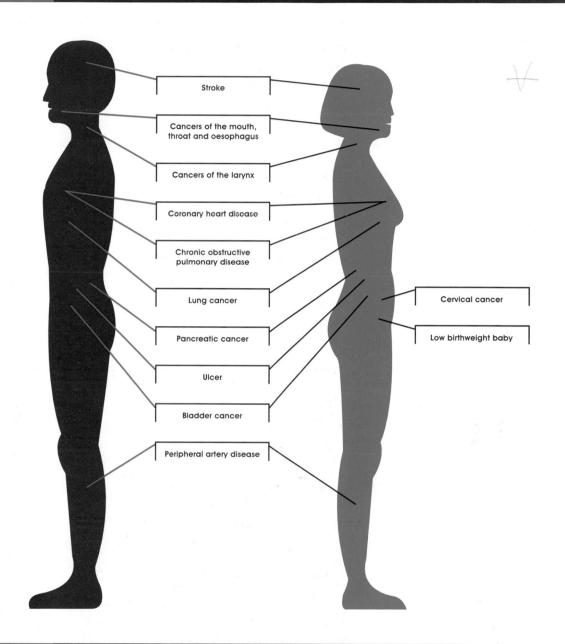

- Stroke
- Cancers of the mouth, throat and oesophagus
- Cancers of the larynx
- Coronary heart disease
- Chronic obstructive pulmonary disease
- Lung cancer
- Pancreatic cancer
- Ulcer
- Bladder cancer
- Peripheral artery disease
- Cervical cancer
- Low birthweight baby

It has been estimated that for every 1,000 young smokers, one will be murdered, six will be killed in a road accident and 250 will die before their time because they smoke[21].

2.21 <u>Some</u> smokers do live long lives but the odds are still heavily stacked against smokers. In 1996 28% of boys aged 15 and 33% of girls aged 15 smoked regularly and these figures are rising.

Complementary Strategies
- smoking
- alcohol
- teenage conceptions
- HIV/AIDS
- drugs

2.22 And a recent study funded by the European Union estimated that passive smoking kills more than 20,000 people each year in Europe[22]. Because of the terrible toll that smoking takes on health, the Government is preparing a comprehensive strategy on reducing smoking to support *Our Healthier Nation*. This will be published later this year.

Alcohol

2.23 Many people who drink **alcohol** enjoy it and cause no harm to themselves or to others. Whether people drink sensibly can dramatically affect their physical and mental health and that of others. Drinking too much is an important factor in accidents and domestic violence and can impair people's ability to cope with everyday life. It has been estimated that up to 40,000 deaths could be alcohol related and in 1996 15% of fatal road accidents involved alcohol. The Government is preparing a new strategy on alcohol to set out a practical framework for a responsible approach.

Sexual Health

'death rates of babies born to teenage mothers are more than 50% higher than the national average'

2.24 Girls who become pregnant in their early teenage years can harm their own health and their career chances as well as the health of their babies[23]. Teenage girls who have to look after their young babies find that their education suffers. Their ability to get a job is diminished. Poor living standards can result, which in turn lead to problems with their own health in the long term. The death rates of babies born to teenage mothers are more than 50% higher than the national average[24]. The prevention of early teenage conceptions is being addressed through a separate national programme.

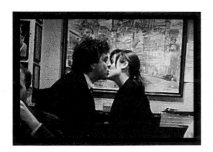

2.25 A safe and responsible approach to sex is an important part of a healthy life. It prevents the spread of sexually transmitted diseases. HIV/AIDS poses particular challenges which continue to require special attention. The Government is preparing a separate strategy to combat the spread of HIV infection and to meet the challenge to services which HIV and AIDS present.

Drugs

2.26 Illegal **drugs** threaten the health of those who take them and are damaging to society and the community[25]. The Government's new Anti-Drugs Coordinator and his deputy are currently reviewing the existing drugs strategy and will advise Ministers in the spring about how it can be improved and strengthened in the future.

Access to High Quality Services

Education

2.27 The Government wants to make sure that children learn at school both the theory and practice of healthy living. And it goes much further than that - **a decent education** gives children the confidence and capacity to make healthier choices and the ability to better themselves and their future families. Poor educational achievement and pregnancy in the early teenage years are closely linked. A range of research studies have suggested that education and particularly nursery education could have an important impact on health in later life[26,27]. The Government has made clear that this means better education for all.

'a decent education gives children the confidence and capacity to make healthier choices'

Health

2.28 **Top quality health services** which genuinely meet people's needs mean that people seek help quickly and get the advice and treatment they need on time. In a fair society there must be fair access to these services for all, regardless of where people live, who they are and how much they earn. But fair access to services is not yet a reality everywhere. For example, some Health Authorities where we would expect to have the greatest need for heart bypasses actually have lower rates for these operations. There is a lower uptake of health checks and breast and cervical cancer screening among some disadvantaged groups. Areas of relatively high deprivation tend to have a relatively low uptake of immunisation. There are particular concerns about the quality of the family doctor service available in some deprived areas. All these aspects of health care bear down hardest on the poorest in our society.

'in a fair society there must be fair access to top quality health services'

Social Services

2.29 **High quality social services** play a vital role in the health of the people that they serve. Decent support for older people, whether at home or in residential care; the protection and care of vulnerable children and young people; support for people with mental health problems; and helping people with disabilities to live more independent lives: health and social care are often one and the same. By protecting the vulnerable, caring for those with problems and supporting people back into independence and dignity, social services have a vital role in fostering better health.

Transport and Leisure

2.30 Finally, good **local transport** planning and affordable **leisure services** make it easier for individuals to be more physically active. Local Authorities in cities such as Leicester, York and Nottingham have

*'leisure services
have a real
influence on
health'*

been among the pioneers in integrated transport policies, combining
measures such as city centre traffic calming and providing park and ride
schemes with initiatives to encourage cycle use. As well as providing
people with healthy transport choices, such schemes have shown
reduced pedestrian casualty rates.

2.31 For example, the City of York has a strategic approach to
transport policy, based on encouraging environmentally sustainable
transport initiatives, including traffic calming and a cycling network.
The city enjoys a relatively high cycling rate of around 20% of all
journeys, while accidents to cyclists and pedestrians have fallen by 33%
and 41% respectively from the mid 1980s to the mid 1990s. Leisure
services which allow people to relax and take a break from the
pressures of day to day life can also have a real influence on health.
Having a place - a public park or gardens, where you can take a walk or
sit, without fear of crime - is a real benefit to health. Sport, rambling
and other leisure opportunities can be equally important.

Inequalities in Health

*'ill health is not
spread evenly
across our society'*

2.32 For many of these factors the extent to which your health is
affected depends on how well off you are, whether you are a man or a
woman, where you were born and brought up and your ethnic
background[1].

2.33 Ill health is not spread evenly across our society. It is concentrated
in particular groups and places. For example, figure 9 shows large
differences in coronary heart disease deaths in people who lived in this
country but who were born elsewhere. Figure 10 shows that children in
the bottom social class are five times more likely to die from an accident
than those in the top social class. Figure 11 shows how deaths from
suicide amongst women have fallen through the 1980s and early 1990s
whereas such deaths amongst young men rose substantially across the
same period.

*'the link between
poverty and ill
health is clear. In
nearly every case
the highest
incidence of
illness is
experienced by
the worst off
social classes'*

2.34 Figure 12 shows that, whereas death rates from lung cancer have
been falling for many years in men, amongst women there was a steady
rise until the beginning of the 1990s. Many diseases occur more
commonly in particular parts of the country. For example, figure 13
shows that more people die of lung cancer in the north of England than
in the south.

2.35 There are many factors that appear to contribute to the differences
in health that people experience. However the link between poverty
and ill health is clear. In nearly every case the highest incidence of
illness is experienced by the worst off social classes. That is why the

Relative Mortality†

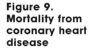

**Figure 9.
Mortality from
coronary heart
disease**

Males, aged 20-69
by selected country
of birth, deaths in
England and Wales
1989-1992

Source: S Wild &
P McKeigue (1997), BMJ
volume 314 (from ONS data).

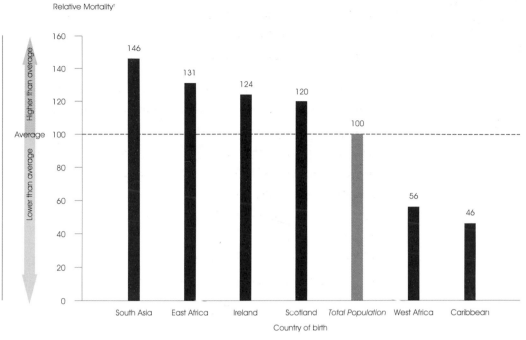

†Standardised Mortality Ratios (SMRs), SMR for England and Wales 1989-1992=100

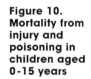

**Figure 10.
Mortality from
injury and
poisoning in
children aged
0-15 years**

By social class
England and Wales
1989-1992

Source: I Roberts & C Power
(1996), BMJ volume 313
(from ONS data).

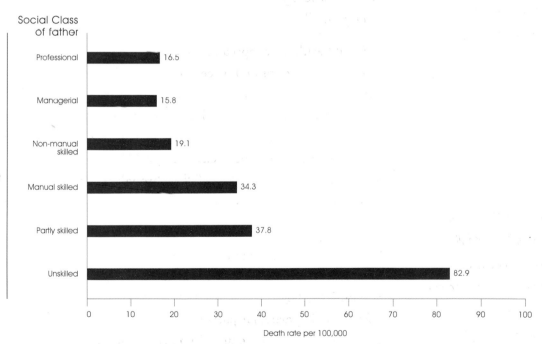

**Figure 11.
Mortality rates*
from suicide and
undetermined
injury**

By age and sex,
England
1969-1996

3 year average rates

*Each age group has
been separately age
standardised, ie adjusted
for differences in the age
structure of the
population.

Source: ONS Mortality
Statistics (ICD E950-E959,
E980-E989 less E988.8).

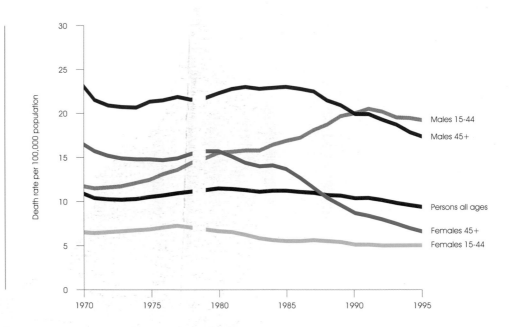

**Figure 12.
Mortality rates from
lung cancer**

By sex, England
1969-1996

3 year average rates

Source: ONS Mortality
Statistics (ICD 162).

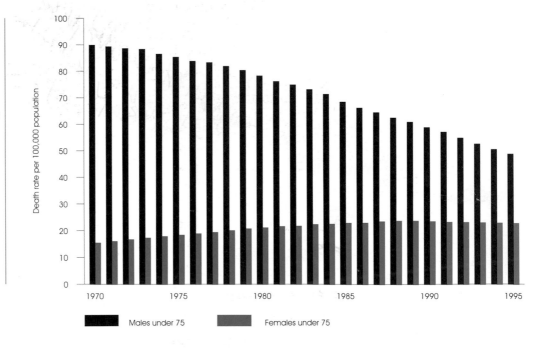

*'Government's
overall
determination to
tackle inequality
and create
opportunity will
reduce the health
gap'*

Government's overall determination to tackle inequality and create
opportunity will reduce the health gap.

2.36 The causes of ill health do not, therefore, rest with individuals on
their own or with Government on its own. They are shared by society.
Chapter Three sets out a new way forward to pull together all who have
a part to play in tackling poor health and health inequalities.

**Figure 13.
Mortality rates
from lung cancer**

By Regional Office
Area, males aged
under 75, England
1996

Age Standardised Mortality
Rate per 100,000.

Source: Public Health
Common Data Set 1997
(from ONS data).

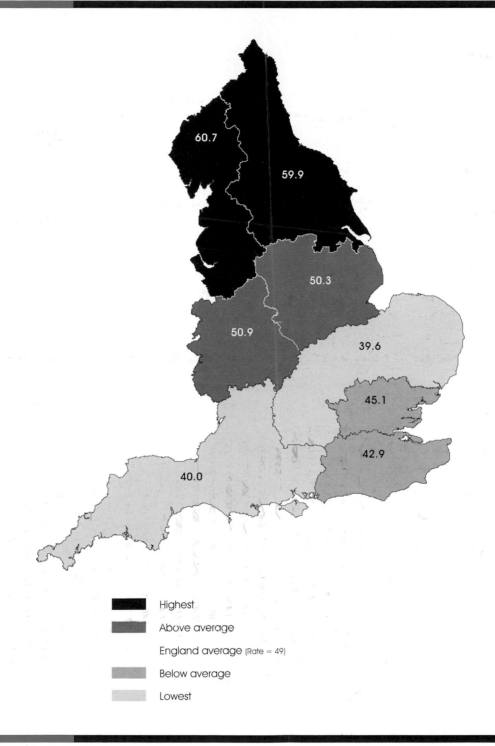

Highest

Above average

England average (Rate = 49)

Below average

Lowest

'the causes of ill
health do not rest
with individuals on
their own or with
Government on its
own'

A Contract
for Health

New Public Health

3.1   In the past, efforts to improve health have been too much about blame. Individuals were to blame for failing to listen to well-intentioned but misdirected health advice. Or the Government was blamed for failing to embrace grand plans for social engineering which would make people healthier automatically.

3.2   In the past, arguments about health ranged between two extremes - individual victim blaming on the one hand and nanny state social engineering on the other. The broad majority who just wanted a normal healthy life for themselves and their families were ignored.

3.3   In a modern country these old positions must become obsolete. Health is not about blame, but about opportunity and responsibility. Everyone has a part to play - Government, national organisations, local services, communities, families and individuals. *Our Healthier Nation* sets out a third way of tackling the problems of ill health that our country faces.

3.4   Individuals on their own can find it hard to make a difference. But with help from their families and support, when needed, from the community and local agencies they can make real changes. Local agencies need central Government to provide leadership and put in

'Our Healthier Nation sets out a third way between the old extremes of individual victim blaming on the one hand and nanny state social engineering on the other'

place the national building blocks and support. Without individuals, families and communities working together, Government achievements will be limited.

3.5   The new approach to public health also means finding more effective ways of using scarce resources, working together to maximise the impact of what we do and recognising the health benefits of investment in other areas. There are substantial additional resources for those elements of our strategy for health which are clearly associated with the promotion of good health - £300 million in the United Kingdom for Healthy Living Centres alone, and additional resources for the Healthy Schools Initiative. But it is the investment of time and resources such as the £5 billion Welfare to Work programme, the establishment of the National Minimum Wage and the reform of our welfare system to help support people back to independence which will be the most significant contributions to the strategy. The Government's Comprehensive Spending Review is considering the health implications of many Government policies and this work will be used to take forward the proposals in this Green Paper later this year.

'help support people back to independence'

A Contract for Health

3.6   To help bring the nation together in a concerted and coordinated drive against poor health, the Government proposes **a national contract for better health**. The contract sets out our mutual responsibilities for improving health in the areas where we can make most progress towards our overall aims of reducing the number of early deaths, increasing the length of our healthy lives and tackling inequalities in health.

'mutual responsibilities for improving health'

3.7   The national contract recognises that the Government can create the climate for our health to be improved. It pledges to deliver key economic and social policies. It places requirements on local services to make progress in improving the public's health.

3.8   But for *Our Healthier Nation* to succeed it must engage everyone with a contribution to make to the national contract. The contract will only work if everyone plays their part, and if everyone is committed to fulfilling their responsibilities.

3.9   This is our new contract for health:

A Contract for Health

Government and National Players can:	Local Players and Communities can:	People can:
Provide national coordination and leadership.	Provide leadership for local health strategies by developing and implementing Health Improvement Programmes.	Take responsibility for their own health and make healthier choices about their lifestyle.
Ensure that policy making across Government takes full account of health and is well informed by research and the best expertise available.	Work in partnerships to improve the health of local people and tackle the root causes of ill health.	Ensure their own actions do not harm the health of others.
Work with other countries for international cooperation to improve health.	Plan and provide high quality services to everyone who needs them.	Take opportunities to better their lives and their families' lives, through education, training and employment.
Assess risks and communicate those risks clearly to the public.		
Ensure that the public and others have the information they need to improve their health.		
Regulate and legislate where necessary.		
Tackle the root causes of ill health.		

3.10 Provisional national contracts for each of the four national priority areas are set out in Chapter Four. So the proposed framework for the national strategy will be:

Our Healthier Nation - Two Key Aims

- *to improve the health of the population as a whole by increasing the length of people's lives and the number of years people spend free from illness.*

- *to improve the health of the worst off in society and to narrow the health gap.*

A National Contract for Health

Four Priority Areas
- *Heart Disease and Stroke*
- *Accidents*
- *Cancer*
- *Mental Health*

A National Target for each of the Four Priority Areas

A National Contract for each of the Four Priority Areas

What Government and National Organisations Can Do

Leadership and Coordinated Government

3.11 To deliver their part in each of the four national contracts, a range of Government Departments will need to work together. The Government has already taken two key steps to ensure that health is a central theme of Government policy.

'coordination of health policy across Government'

- **First**, for the first time ever in England the Government has appointed a Minister for Public Health to ensure coordination of health policy across Government, not just in the Department of Health. The Government has set up a dedicated Cabinet Committee of Ministers from twelve different Departments, to drive the policy across Government.

- **Second**, the Government will apply health impact assessments to its relevant key policies, so that when they are being developed and implemented, the consequences of those policies for our health is considered. The Department of Health has already published guidance, called *Policy Appraisal and Health*, and if necessary this guidance will be revised in the light of experience.

3.12 The Chief Medical Officer is leading a project on public health at local, regional and national levels. One aim is to ensure that the public health function can play a full part in *Our Healthier Nation*. Emerging findings suggest that there is a wide range of expertise and enthusiasm in the public health function. But to build on this, we need:

- better partnership between Local and Health Authorities;

- greater impact from independent public health reports and a stronger role for Local Authorities in improving health;

- greater public involvement, in identifying health problems, developing local strategies to improve health and local community action;

- a stronger national network of experts and interested bodies.

3.13 Expertise in public health needs to be strengthened in all sectors. Developing education and training for the workforce must be a priority. Refocusing research and development on public health issues, rather than just health care, will also be important.

'stronger role for Local Authorities'

'public health needs to be strengthened'

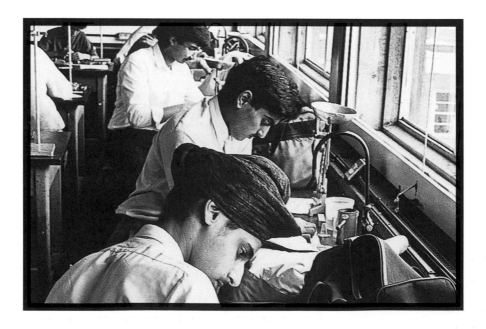

3.14 As a signal of our commitment to the public health function the Government has decided to exempt public health professionals from the

definition of Health Authority management costs, so that our efforts to
curb bureaucracy in the NHS do not create a perverse incentive to
weaken public health expertise at local level. Public health is a long
term investment, not an administrative overhead.

3.15 The regional arms of Government will also have important roles in
the strategy. Government Offices for the Regions coordinate the main
Government programmes such as housing, planning, transport, training
and investment in industry. The Regional Offices of the NHS
Executive, with their Regional Directors of Public Health, oversee the
work of the NHS locally. Working together these bodies should ensure
that the potential of all Government programmes to support the health
strategy is fully exploited.

International Role

3.16 The Government also has an important **international role** to play
in delivering the national contracts. Just as we were able to play an
important role in securing tougher environmental action at the Kyoto
international Environment Summit, we will speak with a strong voice
for the United Kingdom in the European Union, so that European
policies are harnessed to the objective of protecting and improving our
health. For example, we will continue to press for stronger
international action to combat the depletion of the ozone layer. And we
will continue to work with the World Health Organisation, at European
and at global level, to play our part in international efforts to improve
health, including the *Health for All* strategy.

*'we will press for
stronger
international
action'*

Informed Government

3.17 Ministers and civil servants alone do not have the expertise and
knowledge to make our strategy a success. *Our Healthier Nation* will
need a great deal of expert advice to ensure that it makes maximum
impact with the resources available. For example, the Government will
need technical advice on monitoring progress and measuring
improvements in health and the Chief Medical Officer's *Our Healthier
Nation* group will bring together experts to assist in monitoring the
national targets and to provide other expert advice. Government will
also need advice on how best to involve the range of non-Government
bodies who can play a part; and it will need support in making the most
of the contribution of the NHS and Local Authorities.

*'special task
forces to
accelerate
action'*

3.18 In the light of responses to this consultation document, the
Government will consider whether to set up special task forces to
accelerate action on these important issues. The Government will also
need to consider what structures need to be established to ensure that

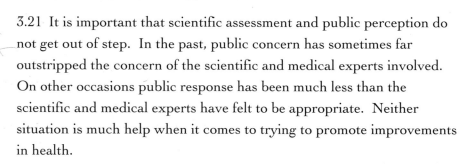

'the assessment and communication of health risks needs to be done better'

all those involved in the national contracts have a voice in the implementation and development of the proposals.

3.19 Good information for policy making and for the public means we will continue to need high quality research and development and a way to ensure that research findings are widely disseminated and acted on. The Government will work across all Departments and with other funders to ensure that research to support *Our Healthier Nation* is put in place.

Assessing and Communicating Risk

3.20 Life is by its nature risky. It is the job of Government to identify risks to health, to assess them, and, where appropriate, either take action to reduce those risks or ensure that people who might be affected are aware of them. The Government believes that both the assessment and communication of health risks needs to be done better. This will require a more thoughtful approach.

3.21 It is important that scientific assessment and public perception do not get out of step. In the past, public concern has sometimes far outstripped the concern of the scientific and medical experts involved. On other occasions public response has been much less than the scientific and medical experts have felt to be appropriate. Neither situation is much help when it comes to trying to promote improvements in health.

3.22 To do this properly the Government must call on the best possible advice from people who command the respect of their professional colleagues. They must also be seen to have no axe to grind. But that isn't the end of the story.

'the public is entitled to know what the odds are so that individuals can make their own judgments'

3.23 The public is entitled to know what the odds are so that individuals can make their own judgments. If they feel that Government is telling them what to do that can actually be counterproductive. For people to be able to make an informed judgment on risk they need to be able to understand and weigh up the evidence. They need to be able to use the information provided. It is very important to communicate the right information in the right way.

3.24 There is no one single way to communicate health information but the Government's strategy will include:

- **Publicity campaigns** The Government will continue to use publicity campaigns on issues such as occupational health, road safety, drink-driving, anti-drugs initiatives, safe sex, and smoking. The Government and the new Food Standards Agency will make sure that protection of the consumer is the first priority in food policy and ensure that we as individuals have the information we need to be able to make informed decisions about what we eat.

- **"*Wired for health*"** With all schools and colleges in the country being linked up electronically on the internet through the National Grid for Learning every young person in the country will have access to the information they need to make responsible decisions about their health. The Department of Health and the Department for Education and Employment will be working together to ensure that young people and their teachers are able to access relevant and appropriate health information at the touch of a button and reach a new web-site, *Wired for Health*, which will link to accurate, clear and credible web-sites on a variety of health issues.

- **Advisory group** The Department for Education and Employment is planning to set up an Advisory Group on Personal, Social and Health Education to advise on the place of this work in schools.

Regulation and Legislation

3.25 Governments have always taken action to legislate or regulate where this was the only way of providing effective protection for the general public or particuler groups such as employees or children. The 1956 Clean Air Act is one example which was necessary to reduce the toll of respiratory disease and death caused by the smogs of the 1950s. Laws to require the wearing of seat belts and to control drinking and driving are examples where changes in social attitudes took place so that public pressure augmented the input of the law.

3.26 Where old threats to health continue or new threats arise we will not hesitate to legislate or regulate if this is judged to be necessary. But we will seek to engage the active support of the people affected rather than resort to coercion or unwarranted intrusion. The contract for health is about partnership and mutual responsibility, about working together to make it easier to be healthy. Regulation and legislation should be the exception, not the rule - a step taken only where voluntary action will not sufficiently protect the public's health.

3.27 That is why the Government has already taken decisive action to secure an end to tobacco advertising and sponsorship, while providing time and help for all sports to allow them to find alternative sources of sponsorship. The Minister for Public Health secured agreement at the European Union Health Council on a framework for an historic Tobacco Advertising Directive, after years of United Kingdom

'a new web-site, *Wired for Health* will link to accurate, clear and credible web-sites on a variety of health issues'

'we will engage the active support of the people... the contract for health is about partnership and mutual responsibility'

'regulation and legislation should be the exception, not the rule'

*'the Government's
main task under
the national
contracts for
health is to tackle
the root causes of
ill health'*

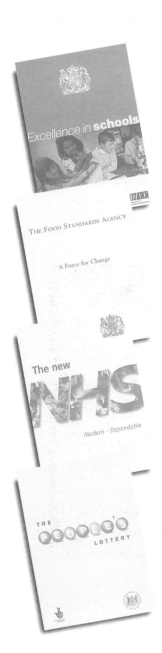

opposition, banning tobacco advertising and sponsorship within the
European Union. But even here legislation alone is not enough to
reduce the prevalence of smoking. A whole range of other actions is
needed against tobacco if the maximum impact is to be achieved from
the advertising ban and if we are to achieve the objective of reducing
the number of children who take up smoking. This will be outlined in
the White Paper on Tobacco to be published later this year.

Tackling the Root Causes of Ill Health

3.28 The Government's main task under the national contracts for
health is to tackle the root causes of ill health. Most of these are social,
economic and environmental. Most of them will therefore be tackled
through those overall Government policies which target help on the
worst off. This means that they will automatically be concentrating on
those people who are ill the most often and who die the soonest, and on
the places with the most deep-seated problems. The national contracts
for health will ensure that we get the most out of the resources and
effort being committed by Government Departments and their local
partners.

3.29 The Government's programme is already well under way. The
Welfare to Work Budget has set in hand an unprecedented programme
to fight **joblessness** with a New Deal for young people, the long term
unemployed and lone parents. Welfare to Work has also been extended
to include people with a disability or a long standing illness. The worst
excesses of **low pay** will be tackled through the National Minimum
Wage. **Social exclusion** will be the subject of a long term, determined
and coordinated Government effort, led by the Prime Minister's new
Social Exclusion Unit. The Government is also working to foster **a new
culture of partnership in business** between management and
employees which will help impact on the problems of stress and
insecurity in work.

3.30 Substantial additional resources - nearly £800 million over two years
- for **decent housing** are being made available under the Government's
Capital Receipts Initiative. This will help Local Authorities to meet
priority housing needs and to improve existing housing. It will help to
carry out repairs and improvements to Local Authority housing, housing
association and private sector housing as well as build new homes.
The money will also be used to carry out energy efficiency improvements
such as insulation, one of the most effective means of tackling health
problems which are linked to cold homes. The Government is
determined that older people should be able to keep warm and keep well
in the winter. It has cut VAT on fuel to 5% and will be making a winter

fuel payment of £20 to five million pensioner households and £50 to 1.7 million pensioner households on income support.

3.31 An **Integrated National Transport Policy**, on which there will be a White Paper later this year, will ensure a healthier environment for all, as part of our commitment to sustainable development. The strategy will tackle congestion and pollution and their damaging consequences, promote cleaner and safer vehicles, and greater use of public transport, cycling and walking. The health benefits will include better air quality, improved levels of fitness, reduced levels of stress and fewer accidents. The Road Safety strategy and targets exercise announced by the Department of Environment, Transport and the Regions in October last year will complement the proposals on accidents in this Green Paper.

3.32 To ensure that initiatives on health and **the environment** have the maximum impact, the Government will ensure that the influence of the environment on health is fully recognised and integrated into major policy initiatives, particularly in the sustainable development strategy and the integrated transport strategy. To improve air quality more effectively and more rapidly, the Government is aiming to produce conclusions on its review of the National Air Quality Strategy by the end of 1998.

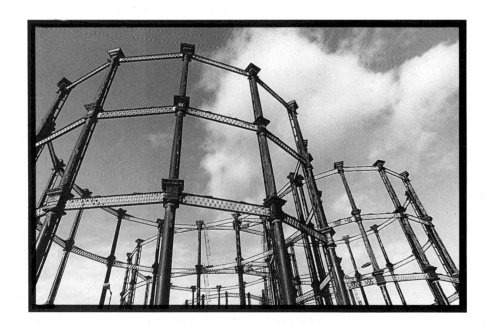

3.33 There is still unacceptably wide inequality in the levels of tooth decay in children. The evidence shows that **fluoridation** of the water supply to the optimum level of one part in a million can substantially reduce the amount of decay in children from similar backgrounds[28]. As a recent example, the water supply in Sandwell in the West Midlands was fluoridated in 1986 and by 1995 the amount of tooth decay there had more than halved. A comparable area without fluoridation saw little change over the same period.

3.34 Current legislation leaves the water industry in the position of deciding whether to agree to local Health Authority requests for new fluoridation schemes. The Government believes this needs to be reviewed but acknowledges the strongly held views on the issue of water fluoridation. It is concerned to explore ways of bridging the gap between those who are opposed to any fluoridation of the water supply and those who believe that only in this way can the children most at risk be protected against the damaging effects of tooth decay. The Government would therefore welcome ideas on how best to test public opinion in particular localities, but it is of the view that fluoridation offers an important and effective method of protecting the population from tooth decay.

3.35 **Tough measures on crime** will help ensure that communities and families are given better opportunities to enjoy healthier lives. The Government wants there to be successful partnerships against crime, such as Neighbourhood Watch schemes across the country. The Home Office's Crime and Disorder Bill will encourage partnerships to develop a target-based strategy for tackling local crime and disorder problems. The Home Office has also increased its grant to the Victim Support organisation, to help those who have suffered as a result of crime.

'our reforms to education will be a crucial component of our drive for better health'

3.36 Our reforms to **education** - with nursery education, smaller class sizes and higher standards - will be a crucial component of our drive for better health. This is in addition to a range of other initiatives as set out in the White Paper *Excellence in Schools* and the related Green Paper *Excellence for All Children: Meeting Special Educational Needs*. Schools will have an important role to play in the national contracts for better health. A sound education has been shown in a series of studies to be central to better health and emotional well-being for all, particularly in helping children who are at a disadvantage socially and economically[26,27].

'sport is an excellent way of fostering good health and a healthy lifestyle'

3.37 Our Sport for All policy has been developed in the knowledge that **sport** is an excellent way of fostering good health and a healthy lifestyle. The policy focuses on extending participation in sport through a national strategy which aims to include all sections of the community, regardless of social background, age or ability.

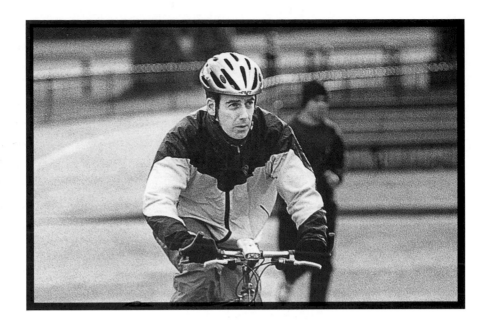

'national
organisations
have important
contributions to
make'

3.38 After completing the consultation on this Green Paper, the
Government will pledge the part it will play in the definitive national
contracts. Other national organisations will also have important
contributions to make. The Confederation of British Industry, the
Trades Union Congress, national voluntary organisations, the Health
Education Authority, the professional Royal Colleges, and many others
can offer their own expertise as well as ensure that their own policies
are health friendly. The Local Government Association, the Chartered
Institute of Housing and Chartered Institute of Environmental Health
can help ensure that their members are well informed about their role in
public health. Other organisations , such as the National Association of
Citizens' Advice Bureaux, the National Federation of Women's
Institutes, the Rotary Club and various sports bodies have extensive
networks of local branches and are very efficient communicators.

'it is people on the
ground, working
locally and
directly with
communities, who
can do most to
make *Our
Healthier Nation*
a reality'

What Local Organisations Can Do

3.39 While Government can set a framework and ensure that the social,
environmental and economic foundations of good health are strong
ones, it is people on the ground, working locally and directly with
communities, who can do most to make *Our Healthier Nation* a reality.
It is within the healthy neighbourhood or the healthy community that
all the local bodies - whether public, private or voluntary - can come
together to improve health. The strategy will be led by Health
Authorities at a local level with action agreed through Health
Improvement Programmes. The strength and effectiveness of
partnerships in driving local action will be key in determining success.

Local Leadership in Health

3.40 *Our Healthier Nation* will set the framework for all of us for improving health. The measures set out in the White Paper on *The new NHS* will improve the NHS's capacity to play its full part in making those improvements happen. Health Authorities will have a stronger, clearer strategic role which will help overcome the fragmentation which characterised the internal market. There will be common goals so that all parts of the health service work together, and in partnership with local government and others.

3.41 When the NHS brings its wide expertise into partnerships with other organisations it can help direct money, staff and services where they are most needed. Health Authorities will have an important **local leadership** role in identifying local health needs and translating *Our Healthier Nation*'s twin aims, priorities, targets and contracts into action. They will lead local alliances to develop the **Health Improvement Programmes** which will set out what each locality will do to help in the national contracts for health. In doing so they will work closely with Local Authorities, well as with other parts of the NHS, local voluntary organisations and businesses.

3.42 To help with the development of these important alliances, Local Authorities will be included in the duty of partnership to be placed on NHS bodies. The Government is considering whether the Local Authority contribution to Health Improvement Programmes can be brought within the best value regime which is being developed for local government. It is vital that both Health and Local Authorities take responsibility for their part in Health Improvement Programmes.

3.43 Health Improvement Programmes will be effective vehicles for making a major and sustained impact on the health problems of every locality in the country. As well as looking at the overall health of the local population, they will also focus action on people who are socially excluded and need the most support in getting back on their feet. Taken together, the Health Improvement Programmes across the country, combined with the Government's role in the national contracts, will form a concerted national programme to improve health and tackle health inequalities. They will be in place by April 1999. We envisage that they will:

- give a clear description of how the national aims, priorities, targets and contracts will be tackled locally;

- set out a range of locally-determined priorities and, targets to address issues and problems which are judged important, with particular emphasis on addressing areas of major health inequality in local communities;

'Health Authorities will have important local leadership roles'

'Local Authorities will be included in the duty of partnership to be placed on NHS bodies'

'Health Improvement Programmes will make a major and sustained impact'

- specify agreed programmes of action to address these national and local health improvement priorities;

- show that the action proposed is based on evidence of what is known to work (from research and best practice reports);

- show what measures of local progress will be used (including those required for national monitoring purposes);

- indicate which local organisations have been involved in drawing up the plan, what their contribution will be and how they will be held to account for delivering it;

- ensure that the plan is easy to understand and accessible to the public;

- be a vehicle for setting strategies for the shaping of local health services.

'Primary Care Groups will be responsible for planning and developing services for smaller populations that will be sensitive to local health needs'

3.44 New Primary Care Groups will be responsible for planning and developing services for smaller populations that will be sensitive to local health needs. Their contribution to drawing up and implementing Health Improvement Programmes will be vital, reflecting the perspective of the local community and building partnerships with key local organisations.

3.45 The Regional Offices of the NHS Executive will agree the plans and monitor the progress of the NHS in achieving the action laid out in the Health Improvement Programmes. A new framework for measuring NHS performance was set out in *The new NHS*. This will make sure that achieving health improvement and fair access to services are central to judging the success of the NHS.

3.46 The NHS contribution to the strategy will be monitored through this new framework. *The new NHS* sets out its six areas:

- **Health Improvement**, which will include performance on the national targets for health;

- **Fair access**, which will ensure that the NHS provides fair access to health services in relation to people's needs, irrespective of geography, class, ethnicity, age or sex;

- **Effective delivery of appropriate healthcare**, which will assess the performance of the NHS in providing care that is effective, appropriate and timely, and complies with agreed standards;

- **Efficiency**, to ensure that the NHS is getting the best value from the money it receives;

- **Patient/Carer experience**, which will focus on the way in which patients view the quality of the treatment and care that they receive, ensuring that the NHS is sensitive to individual needs;

- **Health outcomes of NHS care**, which will focus on the contribution of NHS care to improvements in overall health.

'the public health role of the NHS will be strengthened'

3.47 The tendency to concentrate on the number of patients treated which the internal market brought to the health service means that the responsibility for promoting better health has played second fiddle in recent years. The public health role of the NHS will be strengthened, to ensure that all parts of the health service become more focused on preventing ill health:

- tackling inequality by ensuring services reach areas of greatest need;

- ensuring the right mix of local services;

- holding hospitals and other health providers to account for their contribution to making people healthier;

- ensuring everyone in the NHS accepts responsibility for preventing ill health and not just those people with "health" or "public health" in their job titles.

'the whole range of health professionals, have a role to play'

3.48 The whole NHS will take responsibility for the success of our health strategy and will work together to achieve it. Health Authorities, NHS Trusts, NHS managers and the whole range of health professionals, from school nurses to midwives to dentists to community pharmacists to community nurses to family doctors, all approach health from a different perspective and with different expertise, and all have a role to play.

'we need to develop NHS Trusts as places which actively improve everyone's health'

3.49 The NHS is also the largest employer in the country. It has an important impact on local communities and on the environment. It should set an example as a good employer, showing that it is serious about environmental health and occupational health and safety. We need to develop NHS Trusts as places which actively improve everyone's health - staff, patients and their families, as well as everyone who visits the hospital. This means building on the Health Promoting Hospitals and the Health at Work in the NHS initiatives.

3.50 To do this, the health service needs to make sure that its workforce is properly trained in these issues to allow them to make their full contribution to delivering *Our Healthier Nation*. We need to encourage different professional groups to learn together, and to think about how we plan our workforce to meet the challenges we face.

Local Partnership

3.51 To give first priority to the areas of greatest need, the Government is setting up around ten Health Action Zones as pilot schemes to encourage effective action. They will provide a framework for the NHS, Local Authorities and other partners to work together to achieve progress in addressing the causes of ill health and reducing health inequalities.

'to give first priority to areas of greatest need, the Government is setting up Health Action Zones'

Health Action Zones

The Government is setting up Health Action Zones in England to target health inequalities. Their purpose is to bring together all those contributing to the health of the local population to develop and implement a locally agreed strategy for improving the health of local people. The first wave of around ten Health Action Zones will receive £4 million in 1998/99 and £30 million will be made available in 1999 to Health Authorities for joint spending with Local Authorities and other participating agencies. The intention is to set up a second wave of Health Action Zones in 1999.

Health Action Zones will bring together a partnership of health organisations, including primary care, with Local Authorities, community groups, the voluntary sector and local businesses. They will build on the success of area-based regeneration partnerships and will seek to deliver measurable and sustainable improvements in the health of the public and in the outcomes and quality of services by achieving better integrated treatment and care. They will harness the dynamism of local people and organisations by creating alliances to achieve change.

Health Action Zones are intended to release local energy and innovation, stifled by the NHS internal market and associated fragmentation and bureaucracy, to target specific health issues. Within the national framework, local partners will be encouraged to provide specific ideas and mechanisms. Organisations and groups will be expected to work in partnership with zones delivering support and "investment" against agreed milestones. Building a sustainable capacity from local resources through working in partnership will be vital.

Health Action Zone status should provide added impetus to the task of tackling ill health and reducing inequalities in health. It will provide opportunities for the development of new partnerships to modernise and reshape services in order to improve health outcomes for the local population. The Government wants to see a range of proposals coming forward, offering the opportunity to develop custom built approaches to local problems and challenges.

Health Action Zone status will be long term, spanning a period of five to seven years, recognising the need for a strategic approach. There will need to be evidence of change taking place and of concrete gains for local people throughout that period. It will not be acceptable to plan for the large majority of the benefits to be achieved only at the end of the Health Action Zone's life with few interim benefits.

3.52 In deciding how to implement *Our Healthier Nation* locally and selecting local priorities for action, Health Authorities will not act alone. They must work closely with Local Authorities and with a wide range of other local agencies and organisations which can influence the health of the population.

3.53 **Local Authorities**, with their responsibilities for education, transport, social services, housing and the local environment have the capacity to make a very real impact on the health of the communities that they serve. To reflect this vital role, the Government intends to place on Local Authorities a new duty to promote the economic, social and environmental well-being of their area, working in partnerships with local people, local business and local voluntary organisations. The Government is also considering strengthening the powers for Local Authorities to develop such partnerships. Following consultation, the Government will publish a White Paper on Local Government.

3.54 The pioneering work of Local Authorities over the past decade will be invaluable in securing future improvements in health as part of the promotion of sustainable development . Following the overall Agenda 21 action plan for the next century endorsed at the United Nations Conference on Environment and Development (the "Earth Summit") held in Rio de Janeiro in June 1992 a number of Local Authorities have formulated and are implementing local Agenda 21 strategies. The Prime Minister has called on all Local Authorities to adopt such strategies by the year 2000. To encourage this, the Department of the Environment, Transport and the Regions, the Local Government Association and the Local Government Management Board, have recently published a joint document explaining why Local Agenda 21 strategies are needed and how they can help to deliver other policies, such as local environment and health action plans.

3.55 Many of the environmental factors identified in chapter 2 are raised in the National Environmental Health Action Plan, published in July 1996 and drawn up under the auspices of the World Health Organisation[29]. The Government intends to review the Plan ahead of the next WHO Ministerial Conference on Environment and Health to be held in London in 1999.

3.56 Partnerships between Health Authorities and Local Authorities will be central key components of the local responsibilities in the national contracts for better health. Across the country there are already many good examples of Health and Local Authorities working in partnership, often involving other local agencies as well.

'the pioneering work of Local Authorities over the past decade will be invaluable in securing future improvements in health'

3.57 **Businesses** can bring a new perspective and new skills - such as marketing, project management and communications - to local partnerships as well as considering the health and safety of their own employees.

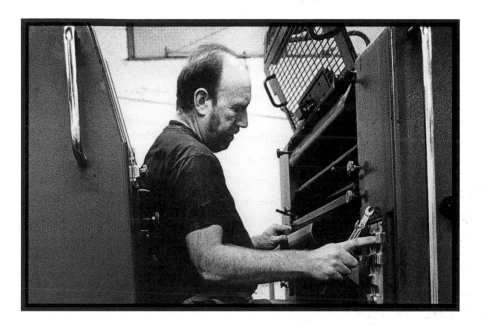

3.58 And the wealth of **voluntary** and **community** bodies brings direct experience and an innovative and flexible approach which can add real dynamism to local projects. Their ability to act as advocates for their members and clients can give them a powerful voice and important influence on local policy making.

3.59 There will need to be effective planning mechanisms to bring all these organisations - the NHS, Local Authorities and other bodies - together in real partnerships, especially where boundaries do not overlap or a single Health Authority relates to several Local Authorities.

3.60 *The new NHS* proposes that Local Authority Chief Executives should attend and participate in meetings of Health Authorities, while other measures could include:

- formal bodies structured on existing models like Drug Action Teams or revitalised Joint Consultative Committees;

- joint appointments by Health Authorities and Local Authorities, including the recruitment of public health specialists to work with Local Authorities;

- joint consultation with local communities to involve local people with the development of plans of both Health and Local Authorities;

- Local Authority participation in Health Authority planning as well as reciprocal arrangements for Health Authority Directors of Public Health to attend relevant meetings of each Local Authority;

- separate health reports for each Local Authority in a Health Authority area;

- Local Authority reports which cover progress on health considerations;

- targeted use of joint funding to tackle health issues.

High Quality Services - Promoting People's Health

3.61 To complement the drive to focus the NHS on the health of the local community, the Government is providing local communities with the means to play their part in *Our Healthier Nation* with legislation to allow £300 million from the National Lottery to be spent on a network of **healthy living centres** across the UK.

'Healthy Living Centres will be the local flagships for health in the community'

3.62 Healthy Living Centres will be the local flagships for health in the community, reaching out to people who have until now been excluded from opportunities for better health, and being powerful catalysts for change in their neighbourhoods. The New Opportunities fund , which will be responsible for administering this money, should be in a position to invite bids for funding towards the end of this year.

3.63 Healthy Living Centres' common purpose will be to improve the health of people of all ages, whatever their capacity and however fit they are. There will be no central blueprint for projects, but there will be quality standards. Bids will be welcomed from a range of organisations. Local voluntary, public and private sectors will be encouraged to work together.

'local voluntary, public and private sectors will be encouraged to work together'

3.64 Healthy Living Centres will be particularly important in the most deprived areas and for those people in poorest health or who find existing health and fitness facilities off-putting or difficult to get to. They will need to cater for the needs of rural communities as well as urban ones.

3.65 Healthy Living Centres will support *Our Healthier Nation*'s aims. They will provide opportunities for local community action to improve health and for individuals to take responsibility for improving their own health. They should be an important means of raising local awareness on issues such as diet, smoking, drinking, drug misuse and physical activity. As far as possible they will be linked to the internet site, *Wired for Health*. The intention is to encourage innovation and energy in developing new and imaginative ways of responding to local needs.

3.66 All projects funded through the lottery are additional to core Government spending. Lottery money complements but does not replace Government initiatives funded through core expenditure. Healthy Living Centres will be additional to existing provision and will neither replace nor undermine what is currently available.

The West End Health Resource Centre

The West End Health Resource Centre, Newcastle is located in the heart of the most deprived area of the city. It provides an integrated approach to improve health, especially for the most vulnerable groups, through:

* health and fitness facilities - including structured programmes for people with chronic conditions;

* community health services, eg physiotherapy and chiropody;

* preventative initiatives;

* information on health and social services, health rights and welfare benefits;

* projects linking arts and health;

* a meeting place and focus for links between local people and statutory agencies.

It is based on a partnership between the voluntary and statutory sectors and local people.

Bromley by Bow Centre, Tower Hamlets

The Bromley by Bow Centre in Tower Hamlets began when a small church congregation opened its building to the local community. It is now an integrated community project on four key areas of health, education, arts and the environment. Current services and activities include:

* a day nursery;

* a community education programme;

* community care services;

* a Bengali outreach project;

* a community cafe;

* an integrated community health care centre;

* transforming a neglected recreation area into an attractive community resource.

The Centre is an independent charitable organisation which receives support from a wide range of sources including private companies, charitable trusts, local Government, the Health Authority and the local NHS Trust. It enjoys extensive support from volunteers.

3.67 And as chapter two discussed, there is a range of other services - education, social, transport, housing, environmental and leisure - which have an important impact on health. For example, the Safe Routes to School initiative, funded by Sustrans, a number of charitable trusts and the Department of Environment, Transport and the Regions has worked with four Local Authorities - York, Leeds, Cumbria and Hampshire - to provide and fund safe routes to schools and colleges for young people.

What Individuals Can Do

3.68   Most of us know that the way that we live affects our chances of a long life and that smoking, drinking, diet and physical activity are important to our health. National and local activity can help provide the environment to encourage healthy choices but it is finally for individuals to choose whether to change their behaviour to a healthier one. For example, in the area of physical activity, Government funds the Sports Council and health education campaigns whilst Local Authorities can provide safe and attractive environments in which to cycle or walk, leisure centres in which to swim or take classes. But it is up to individuals to make use of these facilities.

3.69 Individual responsibility is not only just about our own health. It is also about the example that we set to those around us. The example and boundaries that parents set are central to the health of their children. It is in stable and caring families that children learn the self- confidence to become secure and independent individuals.

3.70 And our own behaviour can affect the health of others more directly. Recent research on passive smoking looked at 37 separate studies of the effects of second-hand smoking and found that there is compelling evidence that breathing other people's tobacco smoke is a cause of lung cancer[30]. And the Royal College of Physicians estimated that symptoms of asthma are twice as common in the children of smokers [31].

Healthy Settings

3.71 As a start, the Government has identified three settings. Each offers the opportunity to focus the drive against health inequalities and improve health overall. Each will be developed as one of three separate initiatives:

- Healthy schools - focusing on children;

- Healthy workplaces - focusing on adults;

'national and local activity can help provide the environment to encourage healthy choices but it is finally for individuals to choose'

• Healthy neighbourhoods - focusing on older people.

3.72 They will involve inter-departmental leadership by Government and partnership at a local level to implement action. In each case we will build on good ideas which are already under way and spread this good practice.

Healthy Schools

3.73 Many of our attitudes to health and the influences on our lives are set in childhood. After the example that the family sets children, education is one of the most important ways of giving children and young people a healthy start in life. This is not just about learning how the body works and how behaviour can affect health. It is also about whether we are able to equip ourselves with the skills and knowledge to make the most of the opportunities life presents.

'many of our attitudes to health and the influences on our lives are set in childhood'

'the healthy schools initiative will raise the awareness of children'

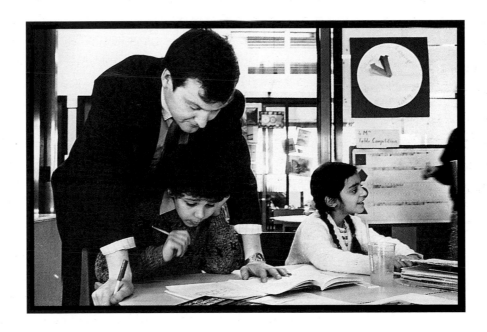

3.74 The box overleaf shows some of the ways in which a healthy school setting can contribute to the national contracts for better health. The approach set out in the contract for health shows how Government leadership, local action and the involvement of children and their parents can achieve improved health, particularly for the poorest children.

3.75 The **healthy schools initiative** will raise the awareness of children as well as teachers, families and local communities to the important opportunities that exist in schools for improving health, particularly the physical and mental health of children and young people. The initiative will include development of parenting skills and the importance of

Healthy Schools		
Government can:	Healthy Schools can:	Pupils and Parents can:
Set high educational standards.	Give children the capacity to make the most of their lives and their future families' lives.	Work together to share responsibility for academic achievement, healthier eating, better exercise, and a responsible attitude to smoking, drugs, alcohol, sex and relationships.
Ensure high quality teaching.	Ensure that children learn about the key influences on their own health.	
Fund safe and healthy school buildings.		
Establish a National Advisory Group on Personal, Social and Health Education.	Provide healthy choices and set nutritional standards for school meals.	Minimise the use of car journeys to and from school.
Establish a healthy schools award scheme.	Ensure that pupils take regular exercise and encourage participation in sport.	
	Create an environment that promotes the emotional well-being of children.	

recognising responsibility to ourselves and to others. It will be a central focus of *Our Healthier Nation* and a key means for improvement in young people's health.

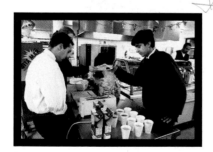

3.76 Whitefield School in North London has set up a breakfast club. It is held from 7.30am to 8.15am each morning. Cereal and milk, two slices of toast and fruit juice is provided for 30p. By the end of the summer term in 1997, 60 breakfasts were provided each day. Initial food supplies came from four local supermarkets - Tesco, Safeway, Waitrose and Marks and Spencer - and the project is now self-supporting. Staff attended, homework became a feature and special deals were done for students with good attendance and punctuality, both of which improved during the project. The club is now funded by the Barnet Education Business Partnership, which is part of the Local Education Authority's collaboration with local firms. Finance is provided on the basis of the number of children on free school meals. Whitefield is also participating in the Barnet Health Promoting Schools initiative which helps schools develop a comprehensive approach to health education and health promotion.

'school nurses and health visitors can play an important part in ensuring that schools, and other places where children gather, keep a clear focus on health'

3.77 School nurses and health visitors can play an important part in ensuring that schools, and other places where children gather, keep a clear focus on health. Other health professionals may also have a role in this. The Government would welcome views on how the health needs of children, both in school and during the pre-school years, can best be met, especially bearing in mind the Government's policy to include more children with special educational needs in mainstream schools.

Healthy Workplaces

3.78 People with a job spend a lot of time at their workplace so a **healthy workplace** is vital to their health. Our aims in developing the healthy workforce are two-fold. First, to improve the overall health of the workforce; and second to ensure that people are protected from the harm to their health that certain jobs can cause. The part that this would play in national contracts might look like this:

'our aims in developing the healthy workforce are to improve the overall health of the workforce; and to ensure that people are protected from the harm to their health that certain jobs can cause'

Healthy Workplaces

Government can:	Employers can:	Employees can:
Set standards of health and safety in the working environment.	Have excellent standards of health and safety management.	Play their part in following health and safety rules and guidelines.
Ensure minimum employment rights to encourage decent and responsible partnerships between staff and managers.	Take measures to reduce stress at work.	Either directly or through trade union safety representatives, work with employers to create a healthy working environment.
Encourage health at work initiatives through the Health and Safety Executive's *Good Health is Good Business* campaign.	Try to create flexible working arrangements that are compatible with employees' home lives and provide childcare facilities.	Support colleagues who have problems or who are disabled.
Through the Health and Safety Commission, publish a consultation paper on a ten-year strategy for occupational health.	Ensure a smoke-free working environment.	Contribute to charitable and social work through work-based voluntary organisations.
	Contribute to and implement the Health and Safety Commission's forth-coming consultation paper on a ten-year strategy for occupational health.	
	Make healthy choices easy for staff, eg provision for cyclists, healthy canteens.	

3.79 Many employers already recognise the benefits of investing in such work. For example, a car manufacturer took advice about product quality testers who were reporting elbow and shoulder pain. A re-design of the equipment cost only £20,000 but increased productivity by 6% and improved the health of the employees. A hospital which introduced an occupational health management approach to lifting and moving patients reduced the working hours lost because of industrial injuries by a third in two years, improving the health of staff, the service to patients and the efficiency of the hospital.

3.80 Efforts to improve health will also have to focus on the needs of people who, for whatever reason, are not covered by changes in the workplace. These include the jobless, older people or those working in the home as carers. The **healthy neighbourhood** will be a particularly important setting to focus effort for tackling inequalities in health. As health and social problems can often be concentrated in small pockets of a locality, when Health Improvement Programmes are being developed they will need to identify those parts of their areas which need particular effort in order to improve the health of the local population. There are already many good initiatives in place, building on healthy cities work or using Single Regeneration Budget monies.

Examples of Healthy Neighbourhood Projects

In 1994 an alliance of voluntary organisations was set up to give a gardening service to older people and disabled people in the Cotmanhay area of Ilkeston. The neighbourhood has a large population of older and disabled people, most of them on low incomes. The alliance involved voluntary organisations, the Local Authority and the Local Health Authorities. The project helps maintain the health of older people by reducing the stress of "not being able to manage like I used to". Regular person-to-person contact helps stop people from becoming socially isolated. The project also aims to help the mental health of the volunteers, building their self-confidence and building new skills and the ability to work and get on with others. So the project helps local people and builds skills in the volunteers to help them get jobs.

And Manchester Health Authority and the Partington Community Enterprise, in partnership with the local branch of the Children's Society have set up a fresh fruit and vegetable co-op run by local volunteers. The Children's Society provide premises from which the co-op is run and a minibus for deliveries or shopping trips for local residents. The co-op is run for the whole community although extra help is focused on older people and disabled people.

3.81 The healthy neighbourhood will often be a particularly important setting for improving the health of older people. The strategy must give older people a better chance of a healthy retirement. If we are to meet our overall ambitions of preventing early deaths, ensuring that people live healthy lives for as long as possible and increasing everyone's chances of a healthy life, then action will have to take account of the needs of people of all ages. There are particular opportunities to improve the health and well-being of older people and they must not be neglected. When we are finalising the national contracts for each priority area, we will ensure that everyone benefits from our health strategy.

'give older people a better chance of a healthy retirement'

A Strategy That Works

3.82 Contracts will only succeed if people feel they have a fair chance of making progress by taking part. So in delivering on aims which are difficult and require long term effort, it is vital that action is based on research and the best knowledge of what works. Hard headed decisions about where to prioritise our efforts will be essential. Good intentions need to be underpinned by a clear focus on effective action and an unsentimental approach to old ways of approaching health which have not delivered the progress that is needed. We shall seek out and publicise examples of effective local projects which show how real progress can be achieved.

'hard headed decisions will be essential'

3.83 In order to ensure a firmer evidence base for our policy, we have set in hand three key initiatives. First the Comprehensive Spending Review is examining all aspects of Government spending to ensure that resources are being used cost effectively. Second, we have commissioned work at the Nuffield Institute for Health in Leeds and the London School of Hygiene and Tropical Medicine to carry out an evaluation of *The Health of The Nation* strategy so that its lessons can be learned. Third, we have established an independent inquiry into the evidence base for action to tackle inequalities in health.

Questions for Consultation

(i)   What are the obstacles to partnerships at local level and how can national Government and local players help to overcome them? Are there good practice examples from which we can learn?

(ii)   Is the overall contract for health comprehensive, or are there other elements which should be added to the national, local and individual roles?

(iii)   How can public health research be strengthened?

(iv)   What task forces might be required to aid implementation of the strategy? What sort of people should be involved in them?

(v)   Have we omitted organisations with a role from this chapter? Are there good practice examples of their contribution?

(vi)   How should opinion on fluoridation be tested in local areas?

(vii)   What further action should Health Improvement Programmes require?

(viii)   How can the Local Authority role in health be strengthened and supported?

(ix)   How can we encourage and foster local community action to improve health? Are there examples of good practice?

(x)   What structures are needed to ensure effective joint planning at local level?

(xi)   What action is needed to make healthy schools, healthy workplaces and healthy neighbourhoods a reality? Are there examples of good practice? What are the obstacles to success and how can these be overcome?

Targets
for Health

Why Set Targets?

4.1   The national contracts for health will need to be clearly focused on areas where we need to make progress on our two key aims:

'to improve the health of the population as a whole and narrow the health gap'

- to improve the health of the population as a whole by increasing the length of people's lives and the number of years people spend free from illness

- to improve the health of the worst off in society and to narrow the health gap.

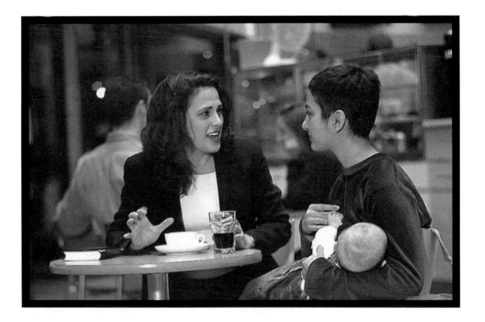

4.2   No one should doubt the seriousness of our approach. In particular, our determination to narrow the health gap between the worst off in society and the better off represents a very substantial challenge. This is because, as our first aim shows, we also want the health of the majority of our people to get better year on year. We will not seek to narrow the health gap by slowing the drive for further progress in improved health amongst the many. So to achieve our vision of narrowing health inequalities we will need to improve the health of the poorest sections of our society very significantly indeed. This will not be easy, nor are there any "quick fix" solutions. We are in this for the long haul.

'we are in this for the long haul...the strategy must be focused and disciplined'

4.3   But operating on too broad a front risks dissipating our energies on too many goals - and achieving none. The strategy must be focused and disciplined. That is why the Government has identified four priority areas:

- **heart disease and stroke,**
- **accidents,**
- **cancer,**
- **mental health.**

4.4   These have been selected because they are significant causes of premature death and poor health, there are marked inequalities in who suffers from them, there is much that can be done to prevent them or to treat them more effectively and because they are real causes of public concern. **To drive the contracts and encourage everyone to take part we propose to set four national targets, one in each of these four priority areas**. By setting targets it is possible to give direction to the strategy, to help everyone involved understand the size of the task we face, to ensure that the right resources are in place and to allow the strategy to be monitored.

4.5   These priority areas, as well as being important in their own right, will also be indicators of overall progress on our two key aims. They are not intended to be a comprehensive measure of all the important factors which contribute to health, but to give a spur to action and an overall indication of the direction and speed of travel.

'contracts for health reflect the full range of social, economic and environmental factors'

4.6   Although the targets themselves will be focused on particular diseases and causes of ill health, the essence of the contracts for health is that they reflect the full range of social, economic and environmental factors which impact on these diseases. Action will be needed in all these areas and it is expected that other health benefits will be seen. For example better access to facilities for physical activity will give a health benefit not only in the area of heart disease but also in prevention of osteoporosis which can cause considerable disability in older people.

4.7   The suggested targets for each of the four priority areas are set out later in this chapter. We believe that they are both **realistic** - not simply wishful thinking with no hope of being reached - and **challenging** - they will require real effort from a wide range of players if they are to be reached.

key Reasons.

Getting the Right Targets

4.8   There are two key reasons for setting a small number of targets. **First**, if everything is to be a priority then nothing will be a priority. So there are tough choices to be made if we are to end stalemates in health and health inequalities that have persisted for many decades. While best efforts on all aspects of health must continue from everyone concerned, hard decisions have to be made if overall health is to improve.

'the rate of improvement for many illnesses can taper off as the easier ways of tackling that illness are implemented'

4.9   So while in consultation we will pay careful attention to arguments for adopting **different** priority areas, **additional** priorities which will dilute our efforts will need a very strong case for inclusion. We need nationally to take responsibility together for the priorities we adopt, so suggestions during consultation for new national priorities will also need to argue their merits against those which have been proposed by showing how they would deliver greater progress on the two key aims of *Our Healthier Nation*.

4.10 Our **second** key reason is that by keeping to a small number of national targets, we will ensure the maximum room for Health Improvement Programmes to set local targets reflecting local priorities.

Getting the Targets Right

4.11 Evidence shows that the rate of improvement for many illnesses can taper off as the easier ways of tackling that illness are implemented. For example, figure 14 overleaf shows that deaths from stroke in people under 65 declined at a fairly steady rate during the 1980s, but in recent years the rate of decline has levelled off.

'Health of the Nation was limited, because of its reluctance to acknowledge the social, economic and environmental causes of ill health'

4.12 The previous health strategy - *Health of the Nation* - included targets. But its vision for health was limited, mainly because of its reluctance to acknowledge the social, economic and environmental causes of ill health. Health and Local Authorities and others achieved some progress on the ground and we recognise and applaud their efforts. But:

- many of the improvements in health over recent years were relatively easily and quickly secured because they related to those in professional and skilled groups who are often responsive to health promotion messages. We want to tackle the much harder task of improving the health of the unskilled and socially excluded as well;

**Figure 14.
Mortality rates† from
Stroke**

England 1969-1996
All persons aged
under 65

3 year average
adjusted rates*

†Rates are calculated using
the European Standard
Population to take account of
differences in age structure.

*The rates for 1984 to 1992
have been adjusted to be on
broadly the same basis as
those for 1969 to 1983 and
1993 to date, using factors
provided by ONS. There is a
small discontinuity between
the years 1978 and 1979 due
to a change in coding from
ICD8 to ICD9 which slightly
affects the comparability of
data.

Source: ONS (ICD 430:438).

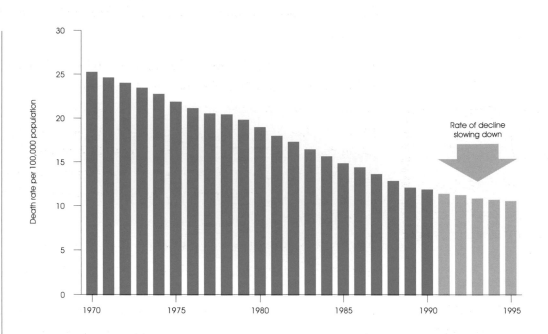

*'international
comparisons give
an idea of the
scope for
improvement but
imply caution for
many diseases'*

- some of the crucial factors leading to a higher risk of heart disease and stroke, such as smoking and obesity, are currently worsening or not improving, making that task even harder. We need to turn these figures around before we can hope to see real health gains;

- it would be highly misleading to assume that even encouraging trends, such as declining numbers of deaths from accidents, are certain to continue. Indeed the evidence points to the need to redouble our combined efforts to reach those groups who have entrenched health problems.

4.13 When formulating our proposed targets, we looked at the experience of comparable countries and their rates of improvement in health. International comparisons give an idea of the scope for improvement, but also help to indicate the timescale over which improvements may be achieved. Those comparisons imply caution for many diseases.

4.14 A number of the suggested targets are for people aged under 65. Many such people are children, breadwinners or responsible for holding a family together. Preventable death and disease in such groups creates suffering well beyond the individual concerned. In addition, it is in these groups that improvements - for example those resulting from changes in lifestyle - are likely to show benefit first. Information about under 65s can act as a sensitive early indicator of progress overall and for all ages. Signs of improvement in targets for the under 65s should in due course reflect real improvements to the health of people who are over 65.

4.15 But the health of people of all ages is vital to overall success and will be centrally monitored as part of the strategy. We know that the policies and programmes set out in *Our Healthier Nation* are relevant to **all** age groups - giving up smoking, regular physical activity and eating healthily is good for everyone - regardless of age. The overall aims of the strategy are to improve health and to reduce inequalities in health for **all** ages. The final national and local contracts for health will reflect this.

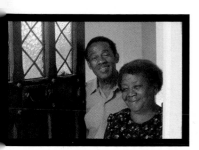

'the policies and programmes set out in **Our Healthier Nation** *are relevant to all age groups'*

4.16 A target year of 2010 is proposed for each of the four targets, because the benefits of the initiatives and activities needed to tackle the determinants of ill health will take several years to be reflected in health improvements. We also intend, after consultation, to set intermediate targets for 2005 so that we can check our overall progress at the mid-point. We would welcome views on whether these time periods are the right ones.

4.17 The Department of Health will continue to fulfil its responsibilities to monitor national trends in health, covering all the main aspects of the country's health and looking at all age groups and sections of the population. We will publish regular updates on progress on *Our Healthier Nation* and progress through Health Improvement Programmes will be monitored on an annual basis.

Targeting Heart Disease and Stroke

4.18 **Heart disease and stroke**, (which, for the purposes of targets, will include all other circulatory diseases) have been selected as a priority area because:

'achievement of our targets would prevent over 15,000 of the approximate 90,000 deaths under age 65 which occur each year'

- they are a major cause of early death, accounting for about 18,000 deaths (a third of all deaths) in men and 7,000 deaths (one fifth of all deaths) in women aged under 65 years [see figure 15 overleaf];

- deaths from coronary heart disease alone account for more than a million years of life lost each year amongst those aged under 75 years;

- these illnesses accounted for an estimated 12% (£3.8 billion) of the total expenditure on health and social services in 1992/93[3]; they also accounted for almost a quarter of total days of certified incapacity in men and 10% in women in the early 1990s;

**Figure 15.
Major causes
of mortality**

Under 65 years
by sex, England
1996

*Deaths occurring at ages
under 28 days are
included in the totals but
are not allocated to a
specific cause of death.
These are therefore
included in "Other". The
major categories
presented in this figure are
those which have been
identified as priority areas
for *Our Healthier Nation*.
All remaining causes of
death have been assigned
to the "Other" category.

Source: ONS Mortality
Statistics.

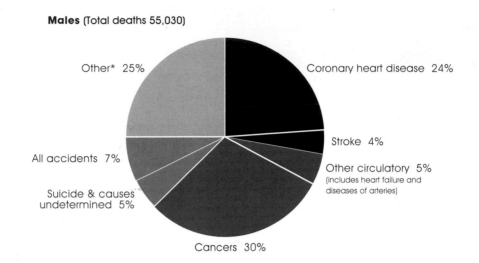

Males (Total deaths 55,030)

Other* 25%

Coronary heart disease 24%

Stroke 4%

Other circulatory 5%
(includes heart failure and
diseases of arteries)

All accidents 7%

Suicide & causes
undetermined 5%

Cancers 30%

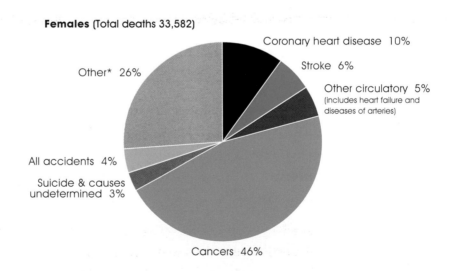

Females (Total deaths 33,582)

Coronary heart disease 10%

Stroke 6%

Other circulatory 5%
(includes heart failure and
diseases of arteries)

Other* 26%

All accidents 4%

Suicide & causes
undetermined 3%

Cancers 46%

**Figure 16.
Mortality from
stroke**

Females, aged
20-69 by selected
country of birth,
deaths in England
and Wales
1989-1992

Source: S Wild &
P McKeigue (1997), BMJ
volume 314 (from ONS data).

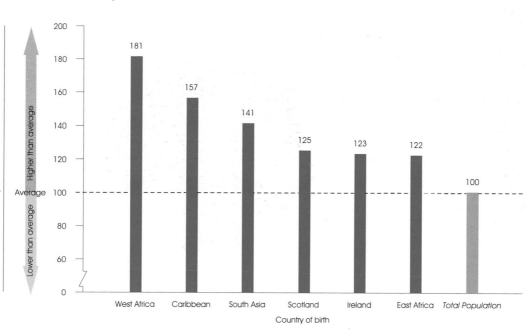

Relative Mortality†

†Standardised Mortality Ratios (SMRs), SMR for England and Wales 1989-1992=100

*'Heart disease
and stroke can
often be
prevented'*

- they limit the ability of people who live with them to enjoy their lives to the full;

- heart disease and stroke can often be prevented;

- they show marked inequalities: for example, women born in West Africa or the Caribbean are over 50% more likely to die of a stroke than other women [see figure 16].

- similarly men of working age in the bottom social class are more than 50% more likely to die from coronary heart disease than men in the overall population [see figure 17 overleaf]; and

- by making headway in tackling their causes we should make progress in other areas, such as cancer and mental health.

**Figure 17.
Mortality from
coronary heart
disease by social
class**

Men, aged 20-64
England and Wales
1991-1993

Source: Drever and
Whitehead (eds), Health
Inequalities, ONS, (1997)
using data from ONS death
registrations and 1991
Census.

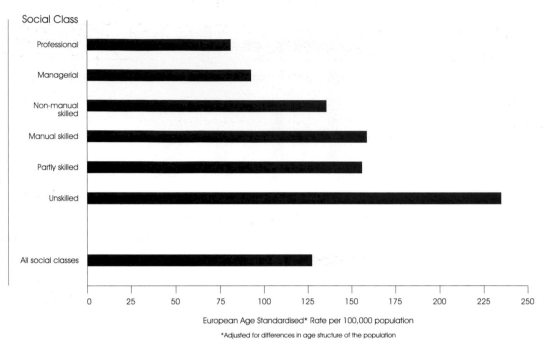

Social Class

European Age Standardised* Rate per 100,000 population

*Adjusted for differences in age structure of the population

**Figure 18.
Mortality from
circulatory diseases**

European Union
aged under 65
circa 1995*

*Data for 1995 except for
Austria 1996; Denmark and
France 1994; Ireland, Italy
and Spain 1993; Belgium
1992.

Source: WHO Health For All
statistical database.

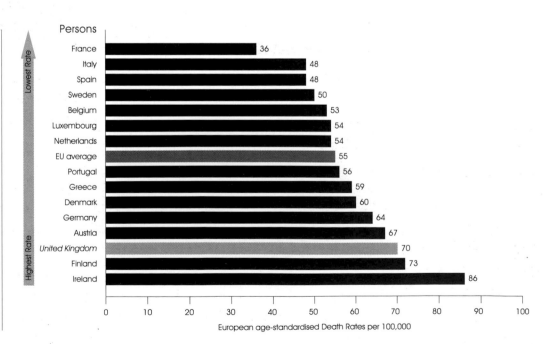

Persons

European age-standardised Death Rates per 100,000

4.19 Death rates from heart disease and stroke have been decreasing for some years in both men and women. Nevertheless, there is considerable scope for further improvement. We, therefore, propose to set a target to **reduce the death rate from heart disease and stroke and related illnesses amongst people under 65 years by at least a further third (33%) by 2010 from a baseline at 1996** (see glossary).

4.20 A target based on the number of people developing heart disease, a stroke or a related condition focuses attention on steps we can all take to prevent such diseases. However, mortality data currently offer the most robust basis on which to set a numerical target. A reduction of this order would, if it had occurred in 1996, have resulted in nearly 8,500 deaths being avoided in this age group.

4.21 Figure 18 shows how this country compares with other European Union countries in respect of death from circulatory disease. The United Kingdom is at present clearly one of the worst performing countries. If we can achieve the proposed target it would bring us to the level which some of the best performing countries currently experience. This represents a major challenge and reflects the Government's determination to deal with the underlying causes of circulatory disease.

4.22 Further progress is not inevitable - in Australia marked reductions in coronary heart disease are now showing signs of slowing and, in this country the rate of reduction in stroke mortality has slowed in recent years. We would welcome views on whether the target suggested strikes the right balance.

4.23 A draft national contract for tackling heart disease and stroke is set out in the table overleaf. It shows some of the key elements which may need to feature in the final contract in the White Paper. As with all the contracts in this Green Paper, they neither exhaustively cover all possible action to tackle heart disease and stroke nor prioritise such actions, as the local component of the contract will need to be agreed by local players in the light of local circumstances. In addition, the Government's role in the contracts will need to be refined in the light of its Comprehensive Spending Review and the responses received in the consultation period. But the contract does show that effective action to reduce the toll of heart disease and stroke will depend on the support and contribution of the range of public, voluntary and private sector players.

A National Contract on Heart Disease and Stroke	Government and National Players can:	Local Players and Communities can:	People can:
Social and Economic	Continue to make smoking cost more through taxation. Tackle joblessness, social exclusion, low educational standards and other factors which make it harder to live a healthier life.	Tackle social exclusion in the community which makes it harder to have a healthy lifestyle. Provide incentives to employees to cycle or walk to work, or leave their cars at home.	Take opportunities to better their lives and their families' lives, through education, training and employment.
Environmental	Encourage employers and others to provide a smoke-free environment for non-smokers.	Through local employers and others, provide a smoke-free environment for non-smokers. Through employers and staff, work in partnership to reduce stress at work. Provide safe cycling and walking routes.	Protect others from second-hand smoke.
Lifestyle	End advertising and promotion of cigarettes. Enforce prohibition of sale of cigarettes to youngsters. Develop Healthy Living Centres. Ensure access to, and availability of, a wide range of foods for a healthy diet. Provide sound information on the health risks of smoking, poor diet and lack of exercise.	Encourage the development of healthy schools and healthy workplaces. Implement an integrated Transport Policy, including a national cycling strategy and measures to make walking more of an option. Target information about a healthy life on groups and areas where people are most at risk.	Stop smoking or cut down, watch what they eat and take regular exercise.
Services	Encourage doctors and nurses and other health professionals to give advice on healthier living. Ensure catering and leisure professionals are trained in healthy eating and physical activity.	Provide help to people who want to stop smoking. Improve access to a variety of affordable food in deprived areas. Provide facilities for physical activity and relaxation and decent transport to help people get to them. Identify those at high risk of heart disease and stroke and provide high quality services.	Learn how to recognise a heart attack and what to do, including resuscitation skills. Have their blood pressure checked regularly. Take medicine as it is prescribed.

Targeting Accidents

4.24 The Government has chosen accidents as a national priority because:

- more than one person every hour died of accidental causes in England during 1996;

- the 1996 Health Survey for England estimated that the annual accident rate, (an "accident" being defined as one sufficiently severe to require medical attention either at hospital or from a family doctor) was 21 for every 100 adult men and 15 for every 100 adult women. Among children aged 2 to 15 it was 31 for every 100 boys and 22 for every 100 girls[32].

- treating injuries costs the NHS in the region of £1.2 billion each year[3];

- accidents are the greatest single threat to life for children and young people;

- accidents, and particularly falls, are a major cause of death and disability in older people;

- childhood injuries are closely linked with social deprivation. Children from poorer backgrounds are five times more likely to die as a result of an accident than children from better off families - and that gap is widening[33];

- there are significant geographical inequalities in accidental deaths amongst young people mainly due to road accidents, and a particular problem in districts which have a significant rural population[35] (see figure 19 overleaf);

- there were nearly a quarter of a million road accident casualties in 1996 of whom more than 3,000 died.

'children from poorer backgrounds are five times more likely to die as a result of an accident than children from better off families'

**Figure 19.
Inequalities in
mortality rates from
accidents in
young people
aged 15-24**

By Health Authority,
1994-1996
10 highest and
10 lowest HAs

Source: Public Health
Common Data Set 1997
(from ONS data).

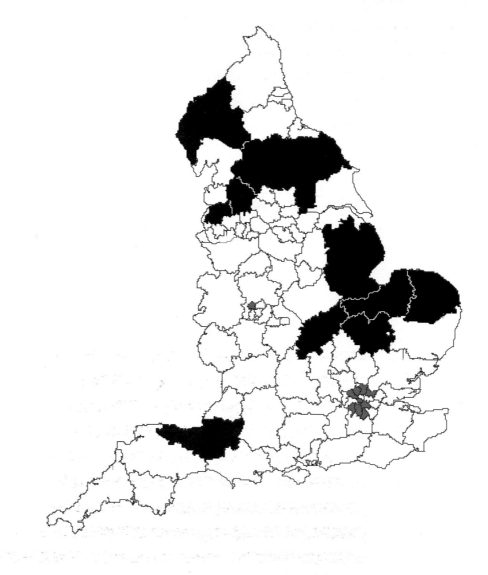

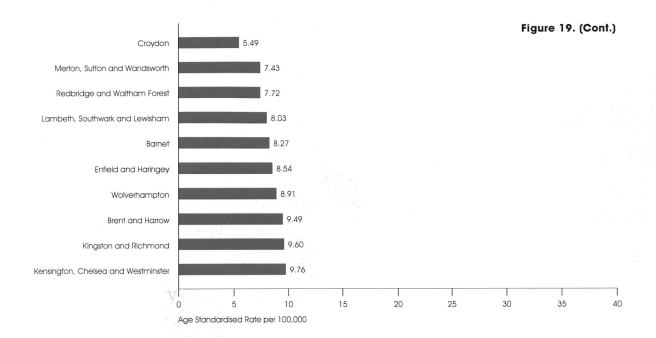

Figure 19. (Cont.)

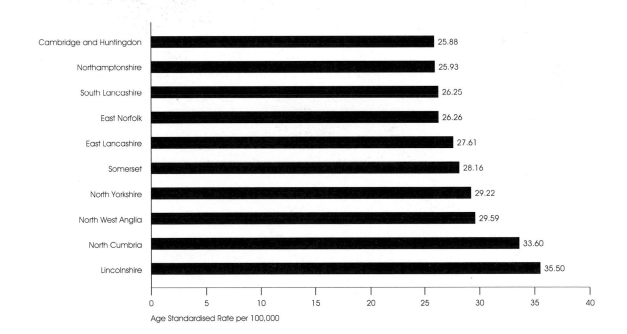

*'many people
suffer prolonged
distress and poor
quality of life as
the result of a
serious accident'*

4.25 Targeting accidents will allow us to focus on our key aims, increasing the number of years of life free from poor health, and tackling inequalities in health.

4.26 It is clearly important that we continue to reduce the number of deaths from accidents. However in addition many people suffer prolonged distress and poor quality of life as the result of a serious accident. We are able to measure the rate of accidents, through the Health Survey for England. We therefore propose to set a target **to reduce the rate of accidents -** here being defined as those which involve a hospital visit or consultation with a family doctor **- by at least a fifth (20%) by 2010, from a baseline at 1996** (see glossary). A reduction of this order, if it had occurred in 1996, when it is estimated that there were nearly ten million such accidents overall, would have resulted in nearly two million of these accidents being avoided.

4.27 The data on non-fatal accidents are not reliable enough to enable us to predict future trends accurately. There is some evidence that rates have slightly increased between the late 1980s and the mid 1990s, although data sources may not be directly comparable. Overall trends in accidents can sometimes mask more worrying trends specific to a particular age group or type of accident. The proposed target is based on the scientific information we have, but given its imprecise nature, we would welcome views on whether the proposed target is challenging but achievable.

4.28 The draft national contract below sets out some of the action needed to meet a national accident target. As with all the contracts, local contributions to the contract will need to be agreed in the light of local circumstances, and the national contribution reviewed in the light of the Government's Comprehensive Spending Review.

A National Contract on Accidents	Government and National Players can:	Local Players and Communities can:	People can:
Social and Economic	Improve areas of deprivation through urban regeneration. Tackle social exclusion and joblessness.	Tackle social exclusion and joblessness in the community.	Take opportunities to combat poverty through education, training and employment.
Environmental	Improve safety of roads. Ensure compliance with seatbelt requirements and other road traffic laws. Help set standards for products and appliances. Promote higher standards of safety management.	Improve facilities for pedestrians and cycle paths. Develop safer routes for schools. Adopt traffic calming and other engineering measures and make roads safer. Work for healthier and safer workplaces. Make playgrounds safe.	Check the safety of appliances and use them correctly. Install smoke alarms. Drive safely. Take part in safety management in the workplace.
Lifestyle	Provide information on how to avoid osteoporosis so that accidents don't lead to broken bones. Run public safety campaigns. Ensure strategies are coordinated across Government Departments and Agencies. Provide information on ways to avoid accidents.	Ensure those in need have aids to prevent accidents, like car seats for babies. Work for whole school approaches to health and safety. Target accident prevention at those most at risk.	Adopt safe behaviour for themselves and their children. Wear cycle helmets. Wear a seatbelt. Not drink and drive. Keep physically fit. Eat a balanced diet which contains enough calcium and vitamin D, take regular exercise and stop smoking to protect themselves from osteoporosis.
Services	Encourage health professionals to give appropriate advice. Ensure professionals are trained in accident prevention.	Provide appropriate treatment to high-risk groups to prevent osteoporosis. Provide child pedestrian and cycling training.	Have regular eye-tests. Know emergency routine.

Targeting Cancer Deaths

4.29 The Government has chosen cancer as a priority area, but recognises that a single target in this area will encompass a wide range of different cancers, with different trends, different causes and different scope for prevention, early detection and treatment.

4.30 Not all cancer deaths are preventable. But many are, either by tackling factors such as diet, smoking or the environment which cause them or by ensuring speedy diagnosis and treatment. *The new NHS White Paper* has committed the health service to ensuring that everyone with suspected cancer will be able to see a specialist within two weeks of their family doctor deciding that they need to be seen urgently. These arrangements will be in place for everyone with suspected breast cancer by April 1999 and for all other cases of suspected cancer by 2000.

4.31 **Cancer deaths** have been chosen as a national target because:

- cancers are amongst the commonest causes of death in this country, accounting for one out of every four deaths - almost 130,000 each year. An even greater percentage of deaths occur at younger ages, one in three deaths under the age of 65 years - a total of nearly 32,000 deaths each year;

- the chance over a lifetime of being diagnosed as having cancer is almost 4 in 10 for men and only marginally less in women;

- cancer is the threat to our health which many of us fear most;

- there is much that can be done to reduce the death rate from cancers. The main causes of cancer deaths are illustrated in figure 20;

- there is very marked social class inequality in who dies from cancer. For example amongst men of working age the most recent figures show that the death rate for all cancers combined was twice as great in unskilled workers as in professionals. This inequality was worse for some types of cancers such as stomach cancer (three times as great in unskilled workers) and particularly lung cancer (four times as great);

- marked geographical inequalities also exist with, for example, death rates from lung cancer being about 20% higher in the north of the country than the national average. Death rates from cancer of the cervix follow a similar geographical pattern, but, by contrast, for malignant melanoma of the skin the highest rates occur in the southernmost parts of the country (see figure 21 overleaf).

'many cancer deaths are preventable either by tackling factors such as diet, smoking or the environment which cause them or by ensuring speedy diagnosis and treatment'

'cancers are amongst the commonest causes of death in this country, accounting for one out of every four deaths'

'there is very marked social class inequality in who dies from cancer'

**Figure 20.
Main causes of
cancer mortality**

By sex, England
1996

Source: ONS Mortality
Statistics.

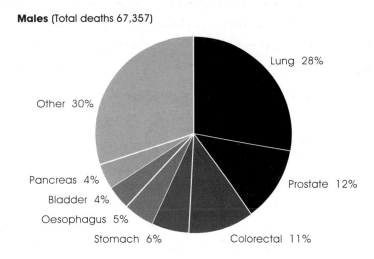

Males (Total deaths 67,357)

Lung 28%

Prostate 12%

Colorectal 11%

Stomach 6%

Oesophagus 5%

Bladder 4%

Pancreas 4%

Other 30%

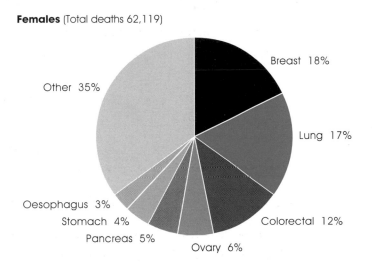

Females (Total deaths 62,119)

Breast 18%

Lung 17%

Colorectal 12%

Ovary 6%

Pancreas 5%

Stomach 4%

Oesophagus 3%

Other 35%

- many of these cancer deaths could be avoided, either by preventing the disease (for example in lung cancer) or by early detection and treatment (for example in breast cancer). Prevention and early diagnosis which focuses particularly on cancers such as lung, breast, cervix, malignant melanoma of the skin, and colorectal cancer could have a major impact on reducing the overall burden from this disease;

- progress in tackling the factors which lead to preventable cancer deaths should help us to make progress in other areas which affect our health.

4.32 We intend to set a single cancer target, **to reduce the death rate from cancer amongst people aged under 65 years by at least a**

**Figure 21.
Inequalities in
mortality rates from
malignant
melanoma**

By Health Authority,
1994-1996
10 highest and
10 lowest HAs

Source: Public Health
Common Data Set 1997
(from ONS data).

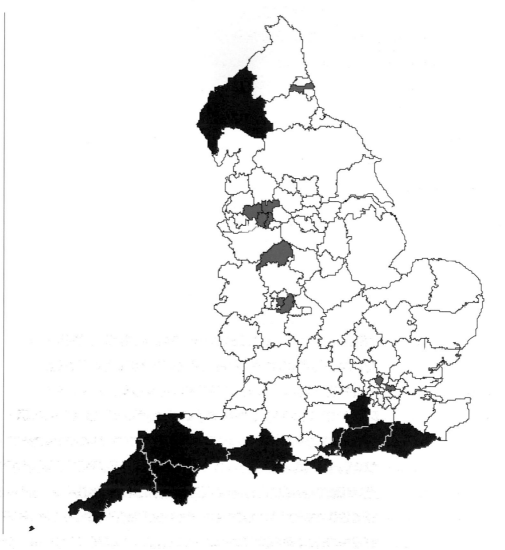

Figure 21. (Cont.)

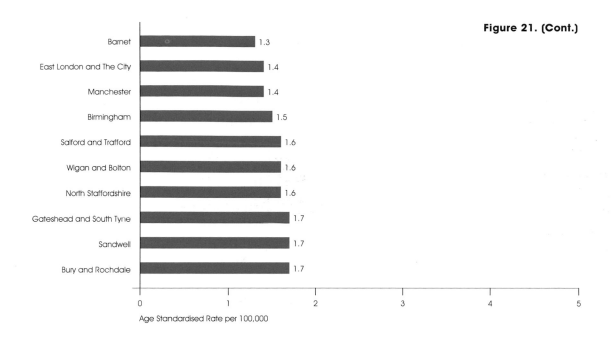

Age Standardised Rate per 100,000

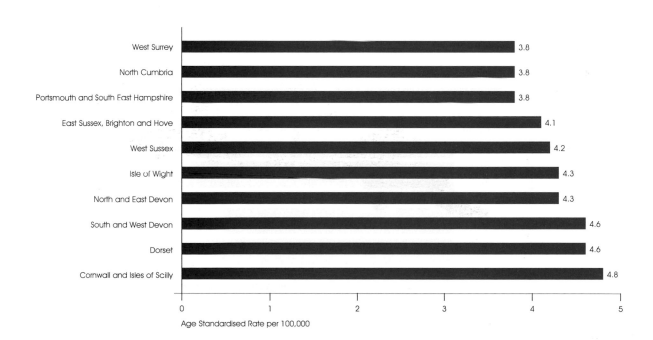

Age Standardised Rate per 100,000

Targeting Mental Health

4.37 The Government proposes to adopt a national target for mental health because:

- the national strategy must reflect more than just the absence of physical disease and be a basis for efforts which acknowledge a more rounded idea of good health;

'mental health is a key component of a healthy active life'

- mental health is a key component of a healthy active life and poor mental health is a risk factor for many physical health problems;

- mental health problems are a major cause of ill health: the 1995 Health Survey for England showed that 20% of women and 14% of men may have had a mental illness[35]; mental disorders accounted for an estimated 17% (more than £5 billion) of total expenditure on health and social services in 1992/93 (the largest single cause)[3] they also accounted for 15% and 26% of days of certified incapacity in the early 1990s in men and women respectively;

- there is evidence of an increase in poor mental health in children and young people over the last three decades, particularly in young people who are socially disadvantaged[36]. Early action in a child's life may improve their health and mental health in later life;

- there are marked inequalities in who suffers most from mental health problems; for example men of working age who are

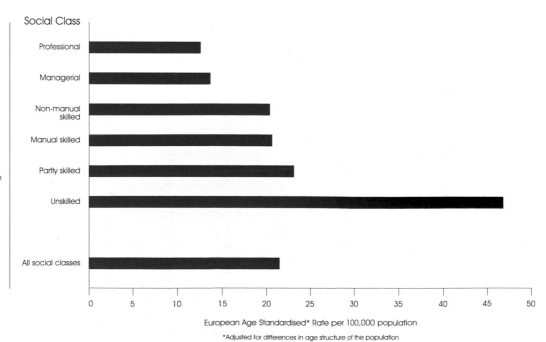

Figure 23. Mortality from suicide by social class

Men, aged 20-64 England and Wales 1991-1993

Source: Drever and Whitehead (eds), Health Inequalities, ONS, (1997) using data from ONS death registrations and 1991 Census.

European Age Standardised* Rate per 100,000 population

*Adjusted for differences in age structure of the population

unskilled workers are more than twice as likely to commit suicide than men in the overall population (see figure 23) and women are more likely to suffer from anxiety, depression, phobias and panic attacks (see figure 24);

**Figure 24.
Prevalence of any
neurotic disorder***

By sex and age,
Great Britain
1993/1994

Adults aged 16-64

*Includes anxiety,
depression, phobias,
panic disorder

Source: ONS Psychiatric
Morbidity Survey Report 1
(1995).

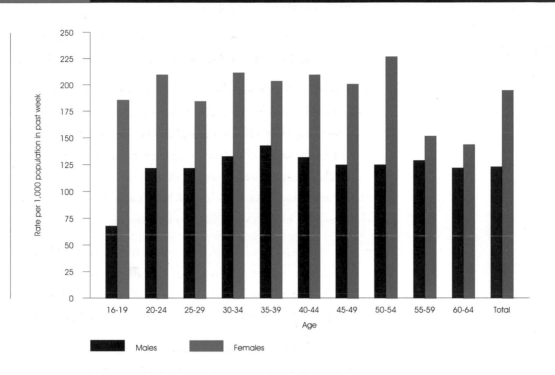

**Figure 25.
Mortality from
suicide**

Females, aged
15-64 by selected
country of birth,
deaths in England
and Wales
1988-1992

Source: V Soni Raleigh
(1996), Ethnicity and
Health 1 (from ONS data).

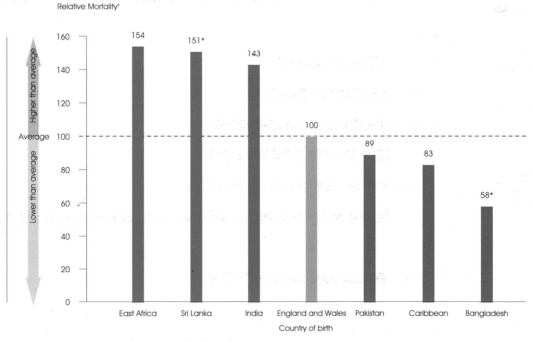

†Standardised Mortality Ratios (SMRs), SMR for England and Wales 1988-1992=100
*Based on a very small number of deaths

- similarly women born in Sri Lanka, India and the East African Commonwealth are approximately 50% more likely to commit suicide than women in the population as a whole (see figure 25);

- suicides are a significant cause of early death, and are responsible each year for nearly half a million years of life lost in those aged under 75 years.

4.38 The causes of poor mental health are complex and the Government would welcome views on how best to monitor progress with a single national target.

4.39 Overall suicide rates have been falling in recent years (though the pattern is different in different population groups such as young men, or women from certain ethnic minority groups). Nevertheless, there is considerable scope for further improvement. A possible target in this area would be **to reduce the death rate from suicide and undetermined injury by at least a further sixth (17%) by 2010, from a baseline at 1996** (see glossary). A reduction of this order, if it had occurred in 1996, would have saved about 800 lives.

4.40 To hit this target will require significant successes in suicide prevention among groups of people in which this is particularly difficult, such as the severely mentally ill.

4.41 An alternative option would be to develop a target which tracked poor mental health rather than mortality and we would welcome views on whether this would be practicable.

4.42 A draft national contract is set out opposite, covering some of the measures that might be taken to meet the national target.

'to hit this target will require significant successes in suicide prevention among groups of people in which this is particularly difficult, such as the severely mentally ill'

A National Contract on Mental Health	Government and National Players can:	Local Players and Communities can:	People can:
Social and Economic	Tackle joblessness, social exclusion and other factors which make it harder to have a healthier lifestyle. Tackle alcohol and drug misuse.	Develop local support networks, eg for recently widowed/bereaved, lone parents, unemployed people and single people. Develop court diversion schemes. Develop job opportunities for people with mental illness. Develop local strategies to support the needs of mentally ill people from black and minority ethnic groups.	Develop parenting skills. Support friends at times of stress - be a good listener. Participate in support networks. Take opportunities to better their lives and their families' lives through education, training and employment.
Environmental	Continue to invest in housing and reduce homelessness. Encourage employers to address workplace stress. Reduce isolation through transport policy. Promote healthy schools. Address levels of mental illness amongst prisoners.	Develop effective housing strategies. Reduce stress in workplace. Improve community safety.	Improve workload management.
Lifestyle	Increase public awareness and understanding of mental health. Reduce access to means of suicide. Support Healthy Living Centres.	Focus on particular high-risk groups, eg young men, people in isolated rural communities. Encourage positive local media reporting. Develop and encourage use of range of leisure facilities.	Use opportunities for relaxation and physical exercise and try to avoid using alcohol/smoking to reduce stress. Increase understanding of what good mental health is.
Services	Develop standards and training for primary care and specialist mental health services. Improve recruitment/ retention of mental health professionals. Identify/advise on effective treatment and care. Develop protocols to guide best practice.	Promote high-quality pre-school education and good mental health in schools and promote educational achievement. Ensure mental health professionals are well trained and supported. Develop a range of comprehensive mental health services for all age groups and alcohol and drug services for young people and adults. Support carers of people with long-term disability and chronic illness. Provide advice on financial problems. Develop culturally sensitive services.	Contribute information to service planners and get involved. Contact services quickly when difficulties start. Increase knowledge about self-help.

Continuity

'the broader nature of these national targets offers additional challenges and opportunities compared with the previous strategy'

4.43 The four national targets in *Our Healthier Nation* build on any success already achieved under *Health of the Nation*. The small number of national targets proposed for *Our Healthier Nation* will offer greater flexibility to focus on particular local health problems and on health inequality. And the broader nature of these national targets offers additional challenges and opportunities compared with the previous strategy. For example:

- the accidents target now addresses a much wider range of accidents, rather than focusing only on fatal accidents;

- the new cancer target includes all cancers, so cancers which were not covered in the earlier strategy will have to be addressed through improved prevention, diagnosis and treatment as part of *Our Healthier Nation*.

Local Priorities and Targets

'health Improvement Programmes will identify additional priorities'

4.44 One reason for limiting the number of national priority areas is to maximise the scope for local flexibility in setting additional local priorities which reflect the particular health problems of local communities.

4.45 In addition to local strategies and local targets for meeting the national targets, Health Improvement Programmes will identify a small number of additional priorities to tackle particular pressing local problems and to reduce health inequalities. For example, although nationally we are concerned that teenage conceptions are damaging the health and social well-being of young mothers and their babies, the incidence is not spread evenly across the country, so setting a national target in this area might be less relevant for some localities. For others it will be a high priority and they will want to target this problem locally.

4.46 The Government is considering how progress on these local targets can be monitored nationally and whether progress on similar problems in different localities can be aggregated nationally.

4.47 Some of the possible local priority areas are set out opposite.

Possible Local Priorities and Targets

Asthma and other respiratory problems - *Asthma is a common condition which can not only lead to death, with over 1,200 dying in 1996, but disrupts education, and is a medical condition often cited by adults as impairing their ability to play a full part in life. Better ways of managing this illness can reduce the health and social problems it can cause.*

Teenage Pregnancy - *Teenage conceptions (particularly for the under 16s) can harm both the health of the mother and the baby and we have high rates compared with the rest of Europe.*

Infant Mortality - *Although trends show improvement, the continuing inequalities in this area mean that it will be an important focus for action in many areas.*

Back Pain, Rheumatism and Arthritis - *In a survey of people over 65 in Great Britain in 1994, 18% said they had longstanding problems with arthritis, 7% said they had "problems with bones" and 4% had back problems.*

Environment - *In areas where housing, homelessness, pollution, or radon are of concern, Health Improvement Programmes may include targets to tackle these influences on health.*

Diabetes - *Diabetes affects more than one in fifty people in the population and can lead to blindness, kidney failure, amputations and heart disease. In addition to prevention efforts, better management of the disease can help to reduce these problems.*

Oral Health - *There are serious inequalities in the levels of tooth decay, both socially and geographically.*

Vulnerable Groups - *In order to address the health needs of specific groups of people whose health is of particular concern, local strategies might address the needs of different minority ethnic groups, homeless people, single parents, socially isolated people, people with learning disabilities, people on low income or refugees.*

4.48 To ensure some continuity, Health Improvement Programmes could, where possible, also include progress against the old health strategy's targets as indicators of progress on the health of the local population.

4.49 In localities where health is already better than suggested by the targets we must safeguard against complacency and ensure that further improvements are still achieved. Areas in this position may need to use benchmarks based on the standards achieved in other countries in order to seek further improvements to the health of their populations, or seek to target particular inequalities in health in their local populations.

Targeting Inequality

4.50 Inequalities in health have worsened in the past two decades. They are a consequence of the widening of social and economic inequalities. While inequalities can worsen in a matter of years, improvements can take much more time, even decades, to achieve. Whilst for some conditions it may be possible to close the gap more quickly, it must be recognised that the overall inequalities in health will only be resolved through long term, sustained and coordinated efforts and not through quick fixes. A sense of realism on the difficulties we face in addressing health inequalities is vital, because false optimism and unreasonable expectations in the short term will only sabotage the long term effort.

4.51 The NHS White Paper signalled that for the first time ever the health strategy will require local policy makers to set targets for reducing health inequalities. The groups and areas who suffer the most from ill health and early death must be a key focus of both local and national activity. Progress on the national targets must not be secured simply by targeting social or ethnic groups whose health problems are more easily tackled. This could have the effect of widening health inequalities. In addition to looking at the health of the whole population, each Health Improvement Programme will need to set out how progress is to be achieved by tackling the health problems of those local neighbourhoods or groups which suffer more from poor health

'for the first time ever the health strategy will require local policy makers to set targets for reducing health inequalities'

The Independent Inquiry into Health Inequalities

The Government has asked Sir Donald Acheson, former Chief Medical Officer, to report on the main trends in health inequalities and to identify the areas of policy which evidence suggests are most likely to make a difference. His report will help the Government in developing the White Paper for *Our Healthier Nation* later this year. The terms of reference of the Inquiry are:

- "To moderate a Department of Health review of the latest available information on inequalities in health, using data from the Office for National Statistics, the Department of Health and elsewhere. The data review would summarise the evidence of inequalities of health and expectation of life in England and identify trends.

- In the light of that evidence, to conduct - within the broad framework of the Government's overall financial strategy - an independent review to identify priority areas for future policy development, which scientific and expert evidence indicates are likely to offer opportunities for Government to develop beneficial, cost effective and affordable interventions to reduce health inequalities.

- The review will report to the Secretary of State for Health. The report will be published and its conclusions, based on evidence, will contribute to the development of a new strategy for health."

than others. Taken together this will mean a pioneering concerted national effort to reduce health inequalities, fully monitored by the Regional Offices of the NHS Executive. We would welcome views on how local inequalities targets can best be monitored centrally.

4.52 The Government will consider the scope for national targets on inequalities in the light of consultation on the Green Paper and the Independent Inquiry into Health Inequalities.

'the Government will consider the scope for national targets on inequalities in the light of consultation on the Green Paper'

Monitoring Progress

4.53 Technical details on monitoring the targets will be published with the White Paper. We will also need to consider ways of monitoring and evaluating local processes to build and share knowledge on the effectiveness of different strategies, techniques and activities.

4.54 In monitoring progress, we will be able to draw on a range of sources of data, such as mortality statistics, cancer registration, hospital episode data, general practitioner data, and various national surveys, for example the Health Survey for England and National Food Survey. The new health strategy will be very broadly based. For the determinants of health, for instance, in addition to the data sources described above, national and local data from, for example, education, employment, transport and the environment will be relevant to the development of the strategy and the monitoring of progress and interpretation of change. We will make full use of sources of comparative information like the Public Health Common Data Set to assist in the presentation of health data in a consistent and comparable form at local level. Other local sources will need to be exploited.

Questions for Consultation

(i)   Are the priority areas, ie heart disease and stroke, accidents, cancer and mental health the right ones on which to focus the strategy?

(ii)   Have the targets been set at the right level?

(iii) Is the approach that is suggested for intermediate targets (ie for 2005) appropriate?

(iv)   What would you add to the draft national contracts on heart disease and stroke, accidents, cancers and mental health? A blank contract is attached.

(v)   How should local inequality targets best be centrally monitored?

(vi)   How should local priorities be determined? On what evidence and by what process?

Your Views on Better Health

'national contracts
for each priority
area will set out
clearly who is
responsible for
delivering
progress'

5.1   The potential for improving health and preventing disease is enormous, but it will require a long term and concerted national effort. By focusing on four national priorities we will concentrate our effort. The national contracts for each priority area will set out clearly who is responsible for delivering progress. With targets to focus our action and indicate our progress, there are real opportunities open to improve our country's health and begin to narrow the gap between the health of the worst off and the best off.

5.2   We must encourage as many people as possible to support this approach and to play their part in achieving its ends. Your views will be taken into account when we finalise it later this year. Some of these questions are set out below but all comments on the strategy will be helpful in getting it right.

Chapter Three: A Contract for Health

(i)   What are the obstacles to partnerships at local level and how can national Government and local players help to overcome them? Are there good practice examples from which we can learn?

(ii)   Is the overall contract for health comprehensive, or are there other elements which should be added to the national, local and individual roles?

(iii)   How can public health research be strengthened?

(iv)   What task forces might be required to aid implementation of the strategy? What sort of people should be involved in them?

(v)   Have we omitted organisations with a role from this chapter? Are there good practice examples of their contribution?

(vi)   How should opinion on fluoridation be tested in local areas?

'your views will be
taken into
account'

(vii) What further action should Health Improvement Programmes require?

(viii) How can the Local Authority role in health be strengthened and supported?

(ix) How can we encourage and foster local community action to improve health? Are there examples of good practice?

(x) What structures are needed to ensure effective joint planning at local level?

(xi) What action is need to make healthy schools, healthy workplaces and healthy neighbourhoods a reality? Are there examples of good practice? What are the obstacles to success and how can these be overcome?

Chapter Four: Targets for Health

(i) Are the priority areas, ie heart disease and stroke, accidents, cancer and mental health the right ones on which to focus the strategy?

(ii) Have the targets been set at the right level?

(iii) Is the approach that is suggested for intermediate targets (i.e. for 2005) appropriate?

(iv) What would you add to the draft national contracts on heart disease and stroke, accidents, cancers and mental health? A blank contract is attached.

(v) How should local inequality targets best be centrally monitored?

(vi) How should local priorities be determined? On what evidence and by what process?

5.3   You can send your responses by detaching and completing the form *Your Views on Better Health* at the end of this Paper, or write to:

> The Health Strategy Unit
> Room 535
> Department of Health
> Wellington House
> 133-155 Waterloo Road
> London SE1 8UG

5.4   This Green Paper can be found on the internet at **http://www.open.gov.uk/doh/ohn/ohnhome.htm** You can also send responses by e-mail to **ohn@doh.gov.uk**

5.5   A summary of this Green Paper is available in English, Hindi, Punjabi, Gujurati, Urdu, Bengali, Chinese, Vietnamese, Greek, Turkish, Somali and Arabic and a taped audio version are available from the **Health Literature Line, 0800 555 777**.

5.6   The closing date for responses to this Green Paper is 30 April 1998.

Glossary and Technical Notes

Proposed National Targets - to reduce mortality from: Heart Disease and Stroke and related illnesses; Cancer; Suicide; and to reduce Accidents.

Target year:
2010 for all four targets.

Baseline year:
Mortality targets: the average of the European age standardised rates for the three years 1995, 1996 and 1997. [NB 1997 data not available until mid-1998, i.e. White Paper stage].
Accident target: the average of the accident rates for the years 1995 and 1996.

Sources of data:
Mortality targets: Office for National Statistics (ONS) mortality statistics from death registrations. Mortality rates are age standardised to allow for changes in the age structure of the population (using the European standard population as defined by the WHO).
Accident target: Estimated "major" accident rates from the Health Survey for England.

Definitions:

Heart Disease and Stroke and related illnesses - includes all circulatory diseases - International Classification of Diseases (ICD) codes 390-459 inclusive.
Age group: under 65.
Target reduction by year 2010 - at least **a further third (33%)**.

Cancer - all malignant neoplasms - ICD codes 140-208 inclusive.
Age group: under 65.
Target reduction by year 2010 - at least **a further fifth (20%)**.

Suicide - suicide and undetermined injury - ICD codes (E950-E959) plus (E980-E989) minus E988.8

Age group: all ages.

Target reduction by year 2010 - at least **a further sixth (17%)**.

Accidents - defined as an accident which is sufficiently severe to require medical attention either at hospital or from a family doctor. Respondents to the Health Survey for England are asked if they had had one or more such accident in the 6 months prior to interview. For children aged 2-15, an adult is asked to respond on their behalf.

Age group: ages 2 and above.

Target reduction by year 2010 - at least **a fifth (20%)**.

Standardised Mortality Ratio (SMR)

The SMR is used to compare mortality rates in different population groupings because it takes account of differences in the age structure of the population. For example, in Figure 5, mortality in different geographical areas of the country is compared with a national standard (SMR for England = 100). If a Health Authority (HA) area has an SMR greater than 100, then the population of that HA has a mortality rate higher than the average for England (after taking account of differences in the age structure of the HA population and the national population).

The **SMR** is calculated as: $\dfrac{\text{Observed number of deaths}}{\text{Expected number of deaths}} \times 100$

The observed number of deaths is the actual number of deaths occurring in the geographical area or subgroup of the population. The expected number is calculated by applying the national age specific mortality rates to the population of the HA area or population subgroup.

References

1. Drever F and Whitehead M (eds). *Health Inequalities*. Office for National Statistics. London: The Stationery Office, 1997 (Series DS, No 15).

2. Confederation of British Industry. *Managing Absence: in sickness and health* London: CBI, 1997.

3. Department of Health. NHS Executive. *Burdens of Disease: a discussion document*. London: Department of Health. 1996.

4. Charlton J and Murphy M (eds) *The Health of Adult Britain 1841-1994*, Vol2. Office for National Statistics. London: The Stationery Office, 1997. (Series DS: No 13).

5. Department of Health. The new NHS: modern, dependable. London: The Stationery Office, 1997. (Session 1997-98; Cm 3807).

6. Marsh A, MacKay S. *Poor Smokers*. London: Policy Studies Institute, 1994 (Research Report; No 771).

7. Stedman JR, Anderson HR, Atkinson RW, Maynard RL. Emergency hospital admissions for respiratory disorders attributable to summer time ozone episodes in Great Britain. *Thorax* 1997; 52 958-963.

8. Department of Health. Committee on the Medical Effects of Air Pollutants. *Quantification of the effects of air pollution on health in the United Kingdom*. London: The Stationery Office, 1998. Chairman: Professor ST Holgate.

9. Sanders CH, Cornish JP. *Dampness: one week's complaints in five Local Authorities in England and Wales*. London: HMSO, 1982. (Building Research Establishments Report).

10. Department of the Environment. *English house condition survey.* London: HMSO, 1993.

11. Luczynska CM. *Risk factors for indoor allergen exposure: health aspects of indoor air: Berzelius Symposium XXVIII.* Stockholm 1994.

12. Platt SD, Martin CJ, Hunt SM, Lewis CW. Damp Housing, mould growth, and symptomatic health state. *BMJ* 1989; 298: 1673-1678.

13. National Radiological Protection Board. *Exposure to radon in UK dwellings.* Chilton: National Radiological Protection Board, 1994. (NRPB-R272).

14. Central Office of Information. *Radon: a guide to reducing levels in your home.* London: Department of the Environment, 1996.

15. Kawachi I, Colditz GA, Ascherio A et al. A prospective study of social networks in relation to total mortality and cardiovascular disease in men in the USA. *J Epidemiol Community Health* 1996; 50: 245-251.

16. Department of Health. *Nutritional aspects of cardiovascular disease : report of the cardiovascular review group.* London: HMSO,1994 (report on health and social subjects; 46).

17. Department of Health. *Dietary reference values for food energy and nutrients for the UK: Report of the panel on dietary reference values.* London HMSO,1991 (Report on health and social subjects; 41)

18. Doll R, Peto R. The causes of cancer: quantitative estimates of avoidable risks of cancer in the United States today. *J. Natl Cancer Inst* 1981; 66: 1191-1308.

19. Health Education Authority. *Smoking kills 330 people every day.* London Health Education Authority 1996 (News release; SMOK/96/0011)

20. Anderson HR, Cook D. Passive smoking and sudden infant death syndrome: review of the epidemiological evidence. *Thorax* 1997; 52: 1003-1009.

21. Peto R, Lopez AD, Boreham J, Thun M, Clarke Heath Jr. *Mortality from smoking in developed countries 1950-2000.* Oxford University Press 1994.

22. Watson, R. Passive smoking is a major threat. *BMJ* 1998; 316: 9.

23. NHS centre for reviews and dissemination. Preventing and reducing the adverse effects of unintended teenage pregnancies: EHCB 1997; 3.

24. Office for National Statistics, Government Statistical Service. Mortality statistics - childhood, Infant and perinatal, England and Wales, 1995. London: The Stationery Office (Series DH3 No 28), 1997.

25. Department of Health Task Force to Review Services for Drug Misusers. *Report of an independent review of drug treatment services in England.* London: Department of Health, 1996.

26. Wadsworth MEJ. Changing social factors and their long term implications for health. *Br Med Bull* 1997; 53: 198-209.

27. Sylva K. Critical periods in childhood learning. Br Med Bull 1997; 53: 185-197.

28. Nugent ZJ, Pitts NB. Patterns of change and results overview 1985/86 - 1995/96 from the British Association for the Study of Community Dentistry co-ordinated survey of cavity prevalence. *Community Dent. Health 1997;* **14**: 30-54.

29. Department of the Environment, Department of Health, *National Environmental Health Action Plan.* London: HMSO, 1996.

30. Hackshaw AK, Law MR, Wald NJ. The accumulated evidence on lung cancer and environmental tobacco smoke. *BMJ* 1997; 315: 980-988.

31. Royal College of Physicians. *Smoking and the young: a report of a working party of the Royal College of Physicians.* London: Royal College of Physicians,1992.

32. Prescott-Clarke P, Primatesta P, eds. *Health Survey for England 1996: findings: a survey carried out on behalf of the Department of Health.* London. The Stationery Office,1998. (series HS; No 6; Vol 1).

33. Roberts I, Power C. Does the decline in child injury mortality vary by social class? A comparison of class specific mortality in 1981 and 1991. BMJ 1996; 313: 784-786.

34. University of Surrey, National Institute of Epidemiology, Department of Health. *Public Health Common Data Set 1996,incorporating Health of the Nation Indicators and population health outcome indicators.* Guildford: University of Surrey. National Institute of Epidemiology, 1997.

35. Prescott-Clarke P, Primatesta P.eds. *Health Survey for England 1995: findings: a survey carried out on behalf of the Department of Health.* London: The Stationery Office, 1997. (Series HS; No5; vol 1).

36. Rutter M, Smith DJ eds. *Psychosocial disorders in young people: time trends and their causes.* New York: John Wiley, 1995.

Your Views on Better Health

We want to hear your views on the plans in this document, and would be grateful if you could spare the time to complete this form and return it to us by **30 April 1998**. If you need more space please continue your comments on a separate piece of paper indicating which question you are answering. Please feel free to photocopy this form.

Please detach and send your completed questionnaire to:
The Health Strategy Unit
Room 535
Department of Health
Wellington House
133-155 Waterloo Road
London SE1 8UG

Alternatively, you can send your responses by e-mail to:
ohn@doh.gov.uk

Important Note: Under the code of practice of open government, any responses will be made available to the public on request, unless respondents indicate that they wish their response to remain confidential.

☐ **Please tick this box if you want your comments to remain confidential**

Questions from Chapter Three

3 (i) What are the obstacles to partnerships at local level and how can national Government and local players help to overcome them? Are there good practice examples from which we can learn?

_____

_____

3 (ii) Is the overall contract for health comprehensive, or are there other elements which should be added to the national, local and individual roles?

_____

_____

3 (iii) How can public health research be strengthened?

_____

_____

3 (iv) What task forces might be required to aid implementation of the strategy? What sort of people should be involved in them?

_____

_____

3 (v) Have we omitted organisations with a role from this chapter? Are there good practice examples of their contribution?

_____

_____

3 (vi) How should opinion on fluoridation be tested in local areas?

_____

_____

3 (vii) What further action should Health Improvement Programmes require?

_____

_____

3 (viii) How can the Local Authority role in health be strengthened and supported?

_____

_____

3 (ix) How can we encourage and foster local community action to improve health? Are there examples of good practice?

_____

_____

3 (x) What structures are needed to ensure effective joint planning at local level?

_____

_____

3 (xi) What action is needed to make healthy schools, healthy workplaces and healthy neighbourhoods a reality? Are there examples of good practice? What are the obstacles to success and how can these be overcome?

_____

_____

Questions from Chapter Four

4 (i) Are the priority areas the right ones on which to focus the strategy?

_____

_____

4 (ii) Have the targets been set at the right level?

_____

_____

4 (iii) Is the approach that is suggested for intermediate targets (ie for 2005) appropriate?

_____

_____

4 (iv) What would you add to the draft national contracts on heart disease and stroke, accidents, cancers and mental health? A blank contract is attached.

_____

_____

4 (v) How should local inequality targets best be centrally monitored?

_____

_____

4 (vi) How should local priorities be determined? On what evidence and by what process?

_____

_____

Q. (M) Personal Details

Title: Mr/Mrs/Ms/Other (please specify) _____

Surname _____

First name(s) _____

Which County/Metropolitan area do you live in?

_____

Is your response a personal one, or are you responding on behalf of an organisation?

☐ Personal   ☐ Organisation

Organisational respondents only:

1) Please state your organisation's name

_____

2) What type of organisation do you represent?

NHS:

☐ Trust

☐ Health Authority

☐ Primary Care provider

☐ Academic

Voluntary/Charity:

☐ Charitable service provider

☐ Other non-statutory group

Local Authority:

☐ Education Department

☐ Environmental Health Department

☐ Social Services Department

☐ Local Authority - Other (please specify department)

_____

☐ Commercial Organisation

(please specify nature of business)

_____

☐ Other (please specify) _____

_____

Which version of the Green Paper do you have?

☐ Full version

☐ Summary version

Where did you obtain your copy of the Green Paper?

☐ Department of Health mailing

☐ Internet

Other source (please specify) _____

_____

☐ Unsure

Where did you learn about the Green Paper?

☐ Newspaper/TV/Radio

☐ Journal

☐ Department of Health Communications

☐ NHS Executive Communications

☐ Internet

☐ Other medium (please specify) _____

_____

What is your overall opinion of the proposals in the Green Paper?

☐ I/we mostly support the proposals

☐ On balance, I/we support the proposals

☐ I/we mostly disagree with the proposals

☐ On balance, I/we disagree with the proposals

Thank you for taking the time to let us know you views. We're sorry that we cannot acknowledge individual responses.

Contract with England to tackle...	Government and National Players can:	Local Players and Communities can:	We all can:
Social and Economic			
Environmental			
Lifestyle			
Services			

Printed in the UK for The Stationery Office Limited on behalf of the
Controller of Her Majesty's Stationery Office
Dd 5067877 2/98 61743 Job No 38637